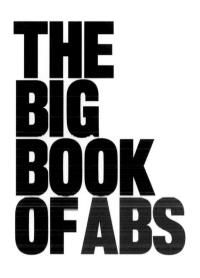

THE BIG BOOK OF ABS

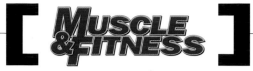

THE BIG BOOK OF ABS

EDITED BY BILL GEIGER, MA

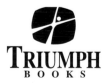

TRIUMPH
B O O K S

ACKNOWLEDGMENTS

Art Direction and Design by Ariel Cepeda
Photo Coordinator is Izabela Berengut
Copy Editors are Kristina Haar and Jennifer Pearson
Production Manager is Lesley K. Johnson
Production Coordinator is Chris Hawkins
Rights and Permissions Researched by Fiona Maynard

Director of Mergers & Acquisitions for American Media is Jonathan Bigham
Group Editorial Director, Muscle & Fitness, Muscle & Fitness Hers and Flex is Peter McGough
Founder/Publisher is Joe Weider
Chairman & CEO is David Pecker
President and COO is John J. Miller

Editorial contributions made by Chris Aceto, Michelle Basta Boubion, NSCA-CPT, Cris Batista, Michael Berg, NSCA-CPT, Frank G. Bottone Jr., MS, R. Daniel Foster, Timothy C. Fritz, CSCS, Ben Kallen, Phil Kaplan, Chris Lockwood, MS, CSCS, Lara McGlashan, MFT, Jennifer Pearson, Carey Rossi, Beth Saltz, MPH, Dan Solomon, Steve Stiefel, MFA, MPW, Jim Stoppani, PhD, Chris Street, MS, CSCS, Debra Wein, MS, RD

Photos by Michael Darter, Ralph DeHaan, Sarah A. Friedman, Bob Gardner, James Georgopoulos, Hacob, John Kelly, Brian Leatart, Blake Little, Ian Logan, Joaquin Palting, Roni Ramos, Robert Reiff, Isabel Snyder, Cory Sorensen, Ian Spanier, Greg Zabilsky

Illustrations by Bryan Allen, Geoffrey Grahn, Ron Guastaferri, Eddie Guy, Bill Rieser

Cover photo courtesy of Robert Reiff

Published in 2007 by Triumph Books, 542 South Dearborn Street, Suite 750, Chicago, IL 60605.

ISBN 978-1-60078-031-8

Printed in China.

Some material contained herein previously published in *Muscle & Fitness* and *Muscle & Fitness Hers* magazines.

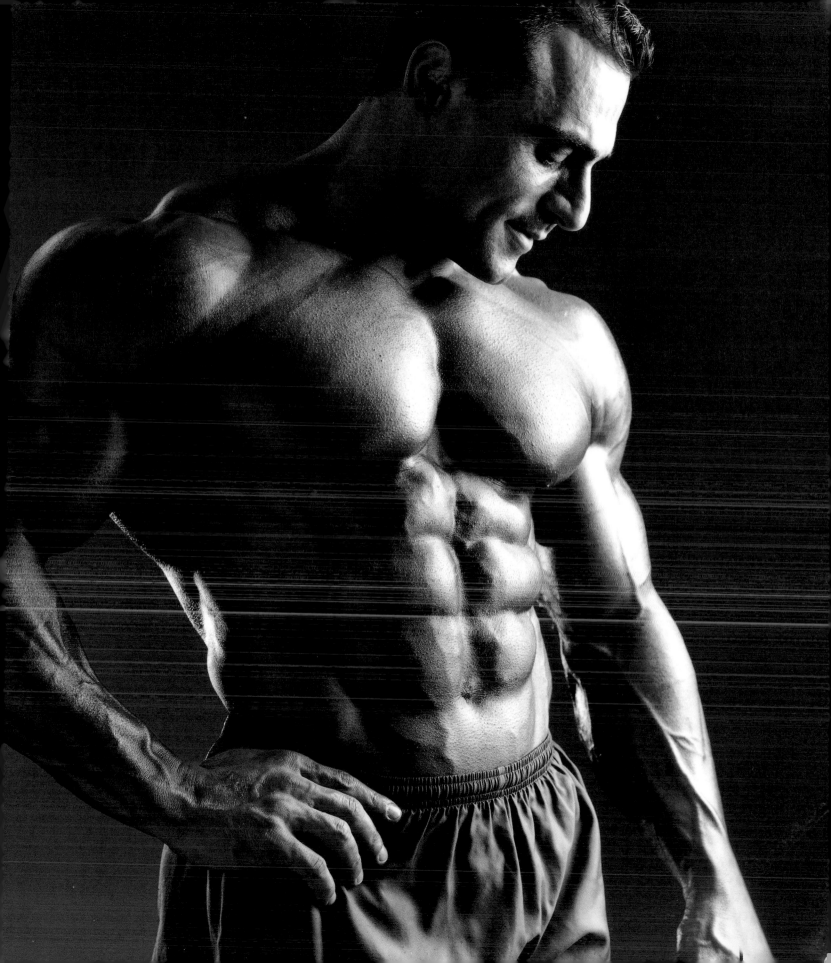

CONTENTS

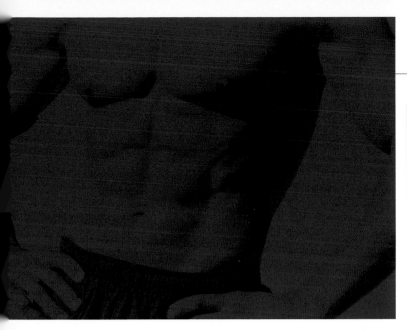

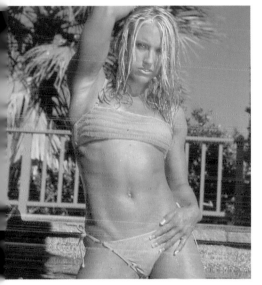

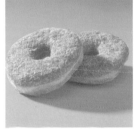

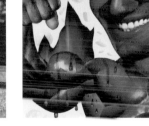

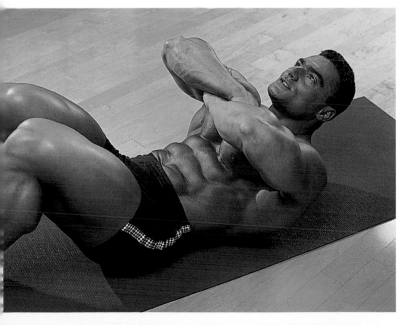

Your First Rep

In the often inexact science of resistance training, a number of roadblocks can limit your progress. You can probably admit to being frustrated by several along your own path to getting fit: missing workouts, trying to catch up on your training all in one day, too many desserts, a late night at the office making you too tired to work out. I remember interviewing one up-and-coming bodybuilder who told me that in his enthusiasm to build the best midsection in the sport, he did 1,500 abdominal crunches every morning and night. That's 3,000 a day! Though this individual finally built the six-pack he so desired, it wasn't without considerable experimentation — not to mention rug burn. Even today, there is a lot of confusion regarding ab training. Should you avoid heavy resistance? Are high reps better for burning the bodyfat that blurs your midsection? Are your hip flexors doing most of the work in a particular move? Is the sit-up a smart exercise choice? How do you focus on your lower abs?

How do you set up an effective routine? Little wonder you can find countless books, videotapes, DVDs and late-night infomercials hawking "the truth" about ab training, all promising flab-free results in minutes a day. If only it was that easy!

The fact is, you can take any number of routes to build a strong and defined midsection, but certain methods are simply better than others. Some people stumble upon what works for them by sheer luck, aided by good genetics and a fast metabolism. Others use trial and error, thinking that some magical combination of exercises will deliver them to six-pack nirvana. In reality, unless you have a very good trainer (which can cost you upward of $1,000 a month) or exceptional DNA, you're going to have to do things the same way as the rest of us — by combining a smart training regimen that gradually progresses over time with a sensible eating plan as well as cardio to help you burn bodyfat. And that lifestyle approach, no matter what anyone tells you, is something you learn to live 24 hours — not just minutes — a day!

This book is an all-inclusive, commonsense approach to laying the groundwork for bringing out your abs in the shortest amount of time possible. No base is left uncovered. Here is a summary of

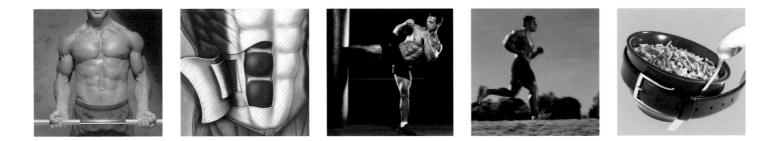

what you'll find in these pages:

>> In chapter 1, you'll find a description of the midsection muscles, along with an overview of the importance of strong abs and some motivational tips to help keep you focused.

>> In chapter 2, you're given a five-week program that's especially suited for beginners and those looking to start with the basics. The workouts build on one another, so each subsequent week's exercises are slightly harder, challenging you as you gain strength. Also included is a cardio program that increases in difficulty over the course of the five weeks, helping you not only burn fat more optimally but making you fitter and healthier as well. In addition, you get a phase-in nutrition plan that allows you to become accustomed to eating right rather than just going cold turkey as you learn all-new nutritional habits.

>> Chapter 3 is a virtual encyclopedia of intermediate and advanced exercises that you can use as your abdominal muscles become stronger, letting you customize your workout for at home or in the gym. The easy-to-follow tips and clear photographs enable you to perform the movements correctly, ensuring faster, injury-free results.

>> Chapter 4 is dedicated to learning how to build an effective ab routine, featuring sample workouts from fitness athletes and bodybuilders with outstanding midsections. Because what works for one person may not work for another, this is a great way to see how an individual customizes his or her routine for the best possible results.

>> In chapter 5, you'll find a comprehensive review of nutrition fundamentals as well as a program on how to vary your carbohydrate intake to optimize fat loss. Fat-loss supplements and a speedy eight-day program to look great, which relies on the same nutritional tools bodybuilders use to peak for a competition, are also presented.

>> Chapter 6 offers four interval-training programs that will help you burn more calories than traditional cardio workouts, speeding up your fat-loss efforts. You'll also find a number of tips on making your at-home cardio routine more effective.

>> Chapter 7 answers some frequently asked questions and provides tried-and-true tips that can make the difference between a program that just works and one that's wildly successful.

Why all the information? Why not just follow a single ab routine? For one, unless you can count yourself among the genetically gifted, getting great abs takes hard work and dedicated effort both inside and outside of the gym. Moreover, what works especially well for one individual might not for another, which is why this book provides so many options from which to choose. Try a number of different exercises and a variety of routines to determine which suit your needs best. Study new movements, ensuring you follow technique guidelines precisely, to better focus the training solely on your abs. Be consistent, be patient and know that you'll reach your goal.

There you have it: Plenty of good reasons to get to work on your midsection today. Fortunately, as your companion you have this book, which includes opinions and sound advice from some of the top scientific experts and professional bodybuilders in the world. Learn from their experience — and their mistakes. In the end, you're more likely to succeed if you follow a plan rather than some random approach. With this book, you have all the tools you need.

BILL GEIGER, MA
EDITOR

[CHAPTER ONE]

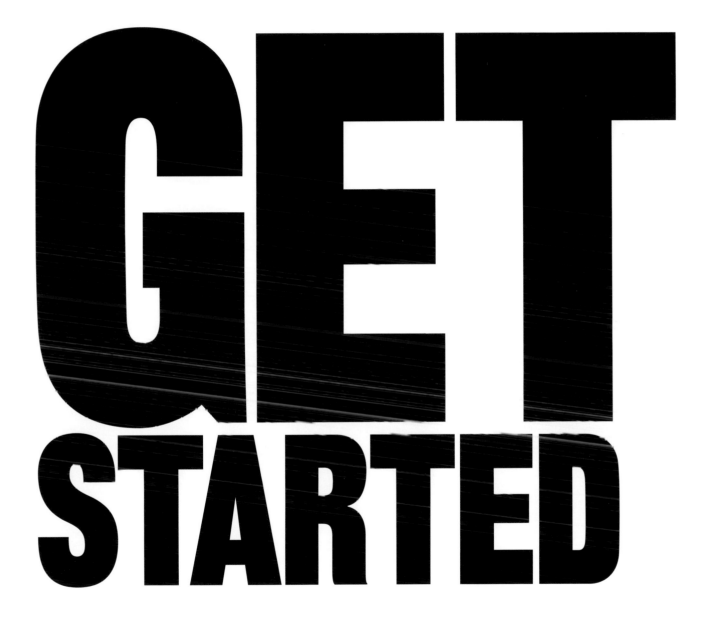

GET
STARTED

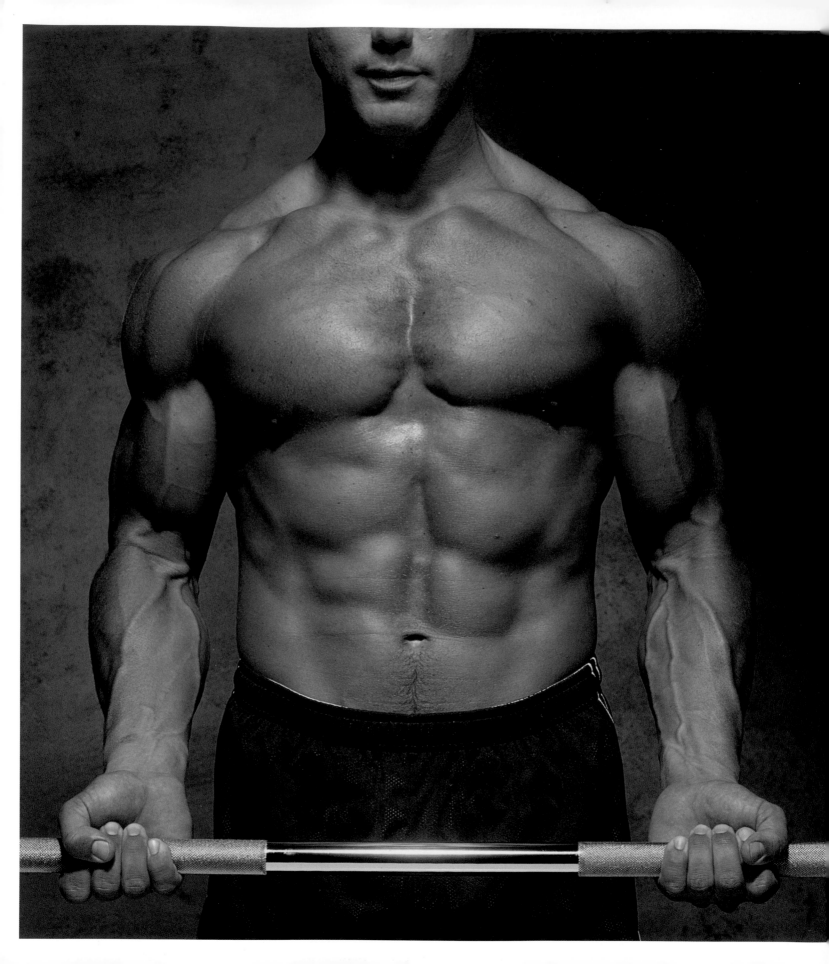

Finding Your Motivation

STRONG ABS ARE CRITICAL, NO MATTER WHAT YOUR REASON FOR WANTING THEM

Admit it — you want a strong and lean set of abs because, well, they look good. Who wouldn't want to peel off his shirt at the beach and show off the hallmark of a great body? In fact, more people say they want a tight six-pack

over any other bodypart. And no wonder: Abdominal fat cells happily inflate to accommodate more food intake, widening your waist inch by inch. Put the blame on one too many Krispy Kremes, but spare a little for your genetics. "There is an inherited component to this kind of fat," explains Madelyn Fernstrom, PhD, director of the University of Pittsburgh Medical Center's Weight Management Center. "But having a genetic predisposition to gain weight doesn't destine you to be obese, only to possibly struggle more with your weight."

Both exercise and a healthy diet are key to abdominal fat loss. "In the long run, it's really hard to cut out enough calories [to lose weight] without exercising," says Fernstrom.

Losing the belly is critical for both your appearance and your health. And we could list a few more reasons you should work your abs — to protect your lower back from pain, improve your posture and to excel at sports are just three of many.

Even if you don't plan to bare your washboard abs, you need strong abdominal muscles for good posture to not just look good but to avoid painful structural problems that can become permanent and possibly debilitating if not corrected in time. Strong abs can bear up to 40% of the weight of the spine. Weak abs provide less internal support for the lower back and let the pelvis tilt back, throwing you out of alignment and straining

your lower back. Out-of-shape abs can force the low-back muscles to work overtime in a variety of activities, often triggering backaches and pain.

If you play sports, even recreationally, strong abs will help your performance — guaranteed. This can be seen in such activities as:
>> When you throw a baseball or football for maximum distance or speed, the main ab muscle, the rectus abdominis, contracts with great force to whip the upper body forward, and the internal and external obliques (located on each side of the rectus abdominis) help rotate the corresponding shoulder forward.
>> When throwing or hitting an opponent in the martial arts, especially judo and some forms of karate, the internal and external obliques help rotate the shoulders to produce force. The rectus abdominis comes into play when throwing an opponent over your body.
>> In hitting sports such as golf, boxing and baseball batting, the internal and external obliques rotate the torso (shoulders). The muscles are most effective when the hips are first rotated forward to stretch the obliques.

Ultimately, individuals bring different motivations to the table — be it health, sports performance or just looking great without a shirt — when they decide to redefine their midsection. Whatever yours is, now you've got a game plan to get you there.

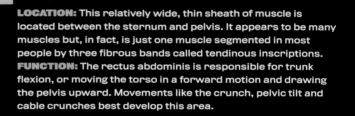

Rectus Abdominis

LOCATION: This relatively wide, thin sheath of muscle is located between the sternum and pelvis. It appears to be many muscles but, in fact, is just one muscle segmented in most people by three fibrous bands called tendinous inscriptions.
FUNCTION: The rectus abdominis is responsible for trunk flexion, or moving the torso in a forward motion and drawing the pelvis upward. Movements like the crunch, pelvic tilt and cable crunches best develop this area.

Transverse Abdominis

LOCATION: Making up the deepest layer in the abs, this thin muscle's fibers run horizontally across the entire abdominal wall.
FUNCTION: The transverse abdominis is primarily involved in abdominal compression, which occurs during forced expiration. Because this muscle doesn't provide much movement, development need not be a primary concern.

Obliques (Internal & External)

LOCATION: Located along both sides of the torso, the obliques are composed of two muscles: The external oblique is the outermost abdominal muscle; the internal oblique is the second layer of abdominal muscle. The external obliques form a V-shape from the pubic bone outward. The internal obliques form an inverted V that runs basically the opposite direction.
FUNCTION: Both the internal and external obliques are responsible for trunk rotation and lateral flexion of the torso.

Anatomy of Your Midsection

A BRIEF TUTORIAL ON THE MUSCLE STRUCTURE OF YOUR ABDOMINAL REGION

The muscle group most commonly referred to as the abs is composed of four separate muscles — the internal and external obliques, the rectus abdominis and the transverse abdominis. These muscles support and assist in moving the torso through various motions, including trunk flexion and rotation. By understanding how each abdominal muscle functions, you'll be able to work your abs properly and in the most efficient manner to develop this bodypart to its full potential.

Abs & Your Genetics

YOUR PARENTS' BODYTYPES MATTER, BUT ANYONE CAN ACHIEVE RESULTS

Two guys follow the same ab workout and diet, but one is ripped and the other is a little soft around the middle. Is that unfortunate guy genetically doomed to a life without the vaunted six-pack?

It's true that every individual has a personal muscle structure that plays a key role in development of his or her midsection. It's also true that everyone adapts a little differently to training, so what works wonders for one person may do very little for another.

Some people are born with the genetic factors necessary for awe-inspiring ab development, and some people have to work much harder for a lot less. But while not everyone can sport a perfect six-pack, just about everyone can build a more pleasing, athletic looking physique with a sensible program.

If you train and train and just can't seem to bring out your abs, the problem could be due to several factors: bodyfat levels, proper exercise selection, even performing the right number of repetitions. The key to maximizing your genetic potential is to determine what rep ranges develop your abs and how to manipulate your diet to drop bodyfat.

We're now learning that having a high amount of bodyfat has a genetic component. We know that the composition of your muscle fibers relates to genetics as well. So do individual hormone levels. Studies have also shown that the ratio of fast- to slow-twitch muscle fibers (something you can't control), along with your sensitivity to insulin, may impact the jiggle around your middle.

So, yes, genetics is a governing factor for success in developing that rock-hard six-pack. Understanding your genetics will enable you to customize your workouts and eating program. If you set goals realistic to your bodytype and stay consistent with your training and diet, you'll find that you can still make vast improvements, no matter what your parents gave you.

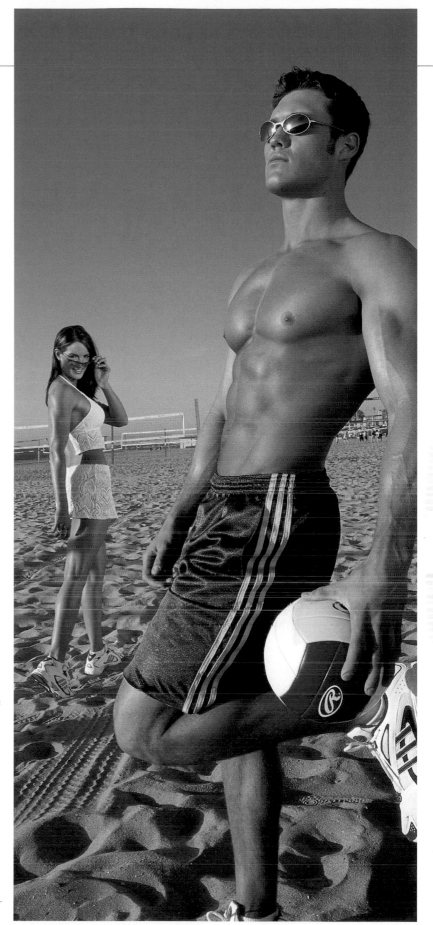

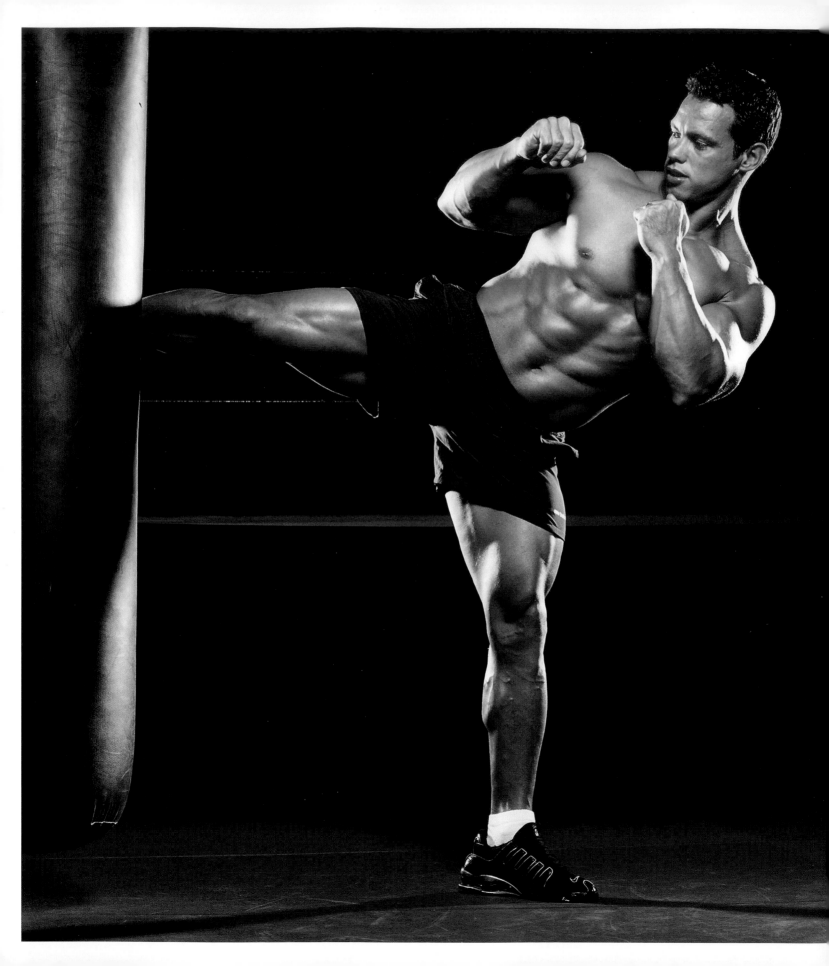

Barrier Busters

21 WAYS TO OVERCOME MENTAL OBSTACLES TO GETTING AND STAYING FIT

We know that lots of things can stand in the way of your desire to get fit and turn regular workouts into a permanent fixture in your life. Fortunately, for each of these problems there are relatively simple solutions. Here are 21 ways to break down the most common mental barriers to a consistent, successful workout program and become the kind of guy who gets fit and stays there.

Fitness Barrier: Missing Motivation

If you're having trouble keeping your fitness plan going, this is most likely issue No. 1. "For most people, motivation is the primary obstacle to beginning and continuing an exercise program," says Jay Kimiecik, associate professor in health promotion at Miami University of Ohio and the author of *The Intrinsic Exerciser*. "In my experience doing research and interviewing 'exercise maintainers,' I've learned that the people who are successful develop a strong enough passion for movement that they overcome the motivational obstacles others fall prey to. You really need to make a connection with the experience you have with moving your body."

[BREAK ON THROUGH]

1 Decide on your goals
Do you want to bring out your six-pack, lose bodyfat, gain muscle, look better, be healthier, live longer, be a stronger competitor in sports — or any combination of those goals? Until someone invents a magic pill, regular exercise is the only clear route to all of them.

2 Learn to enjoy the feeling of exercise
You can learn to take satisfaction from the work your muscles are doing — just as you do when playing any sport — by being aware of the effort you're giving and the progress you're making in the gym. The endorphins don't hurt, either.

3 Focus on the challenge
Working out allows you to learn new skills, progress toward new objectives and gain mastery over your body. After every exercise session, congratulate yourself on achieving something now and taking another step toward your goal.

4 Have fun with your friends
You can make exercise a social event by working out with the guys (or girls). A competitive spirit will likely permeate the group, which will help you work harder and put on muscle quickly. Or you can train separately and get together with your buddies afterward for, say, a post-workout meal.

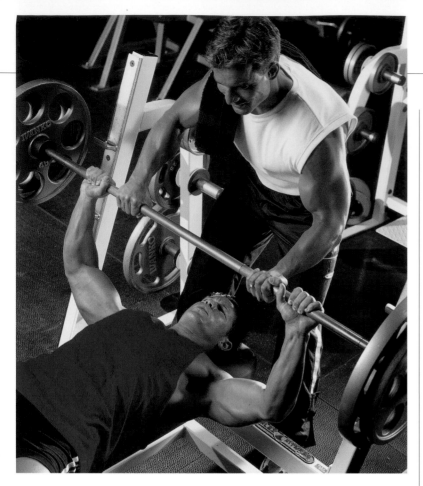

often don't follow through when it turns into a day-to-day task that requires actually doing something about it. But while most individuals start to enjoy working out once they've made it part of their routine, many don't even get that far. "I don't think people really get hooked on exercise until they've done it for a while," says Daniel M. Landers, PhD, regent's professor in the department of kinesiology at Arizona State University (Tempe). The point, then, is to get past those first few months.

[BREAK ON THROUGH]

8) Hold yourself to a time commitment

When you start a new program, promise yourself you absolutely aren't going to quit for three months, the usual length of time it takes to turn your wish into commitment. By then, you'll have started experiencing some physical and psychological benefits, and you're more likely to keep going than you would be if you'd stopped after a month.

9) Create a reward system

Do something that feels good following an exercise session, such as getting a world-class massage. Eventually, the enjoyment that comes from exercising regularly will become a reward in itself. The massage may become part of the ritual, too.

10) Don't get down on yourself

The first time you have an impulse to quit or miss a workout, don't beat yourself up over it. Instead, try to reconnect with the feeling of accomplishment you had when you started working out and the sense of self-mastery that comes from taking steps toward your goals.

QUICKTIP INTO THE PAST

If your workouts are starting to lag or you're thinking about blowing them off, make a list of everything you were doing differently when they were going well — what you were eating, how you were sleeping, what your life was like. Then do whatever you can to re-create those conditions.

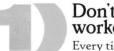

11) Don't let a missed workout spell the end

Every time you miss a session, immediately plan a new one — for the next day, if possible. Remember, it's easier to get back on the mental track by making up one missed workout than it is after missing five of them.

5) Hire a personal trainer to work with you

Even if you only meet with him or her occasionally, a trainer will help you put more into your workouts without injury, and having to pay for the privilege will spur you to keep exercising between sessions. You'll also learn new ways to approach your training — a good thing for preventing the staleness that accompanies doing the same old thing.

6) Pump up your energy

Instead of just dragging yourself to the gym, do something enjoyable to get yourself "up" before your workout, such as listening to fast music or taking a brisk run outdoors.

7) Make it a game

Take up a sport you enjoy and use your training to help you become a more effective competitor. You'll probably discover that gaining strength and stamina is enjoyable for its own sake.

Fitness Barrier: Wanting to Quit

There's a reason health clubs are packed in January and half empty in March: People get excited by the concept of becoming fit, but

12) Go back over your original set of goals

People who bail on a workout program conveniently allow themselves to forget why they started it in the first place. Don't let this happen to you.

13) Think of exercise as a lifelong habit

Don't think of it as an instant cure-all. If you want to be ambulatory at 85, not just have great abs in your 30s, exercise must have a permanent berth in your weekly schedule and be a priority throughout your life.

14) Don't get discouraged

Your progress may seem slow, but no one goes from schlub to hardbody in a couple of months. You'll never get there if you give up now. Plan your growth in increments, and congratulate yourself for the progress you make at every step.

15) Don't let impatience lead to overexercising

If you're tempted to work out too long or too often to speed things up, don't. Overexercising can quickly lead to overtraining syndrome and injury, and it won't make your muscles grow any faster. Keep in mind that rest, recovery and proper nutrition between workouts are the keys to fitness and a great-looking body.

Fitness Barrier: Adhering to an Unfit Lifestyle

Going to the gym for an hour is a great start, but what about the rest of the day? The individuals who are successful in a fitness program and who stick with it over the long haul are the ones who live fit lives. "The more you can get yourself to exercise and the more others around you respond to that, the stronger your 'exercise identity' becomes," says Dean Anderson, PhD, a sports sociologist and a professor in the department of health and human performance at Iowa State University (Ames). "And the more committed you become to thinking of yourself that way, the more likely you are to stick with it."

[BREAK ON THROUGH]

16) Get other people on your side

Let your friends and family know you're working out so they can encourage you to stick with it (and razz you if you don't).

17) Go shopping

Buying all the gym equipment and clothes you need will keep you thinking of yourself as an exerciser — but remember, no spandex. Of course, don't go whole hog on the expense side; start with what you need immediately, then add to it as you progress.

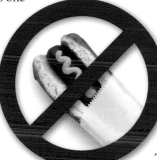

18) Junk the junk food

Stocking your larder with lean protein, fresh produce and complex carbs — beer doesn't qualify — will keep you energized and help you get the greatest benefit from your workouts. It'll also help you think of your body as a temple, not the Temple of Doom.

19) Stop smoking, drinking too much and staying out late

Tobacco destroys your cardiovascular system, drinking dehydrates you and lack of sleep keeps you from producing enough of those muscle-building hormones. But beyond that, when you party every night, you miss out on that great feeling of being fit and healthy that exercise will bring you if you let it.

20) Feel the confidence

When you work out regularly, you end up boosting your self-image. That's not just because you start to look better, but also because you're accomplishing something with visible results every week.

21) Get physical all the time

What's the point of becoming fit if you're still going to hang out on the couch all day? Start discovering the physical benefits of being in good condition, from sports to hiking and camping outdoors to better sex. Once you've learned how much more fun your life can be, you'll never want to go back.

CHAPTER TWO

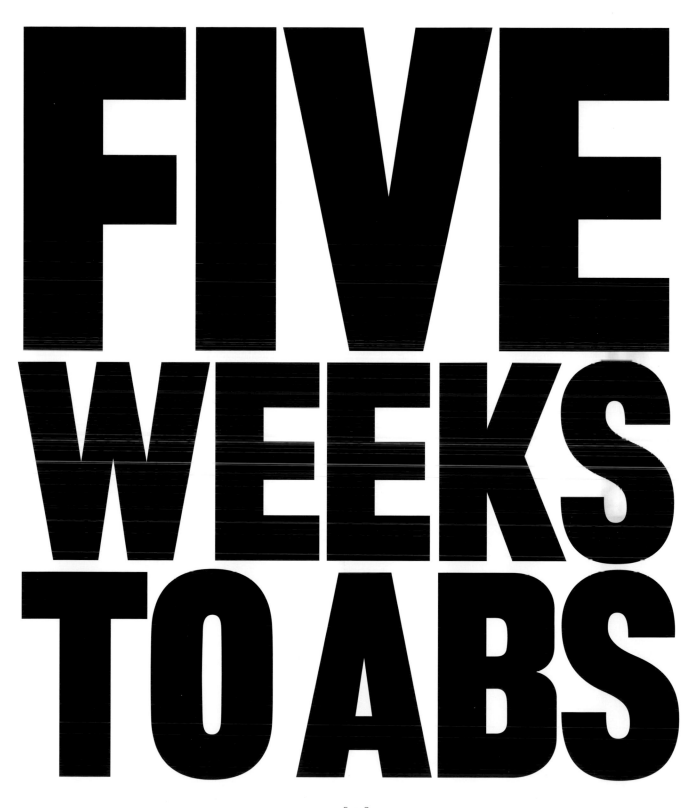

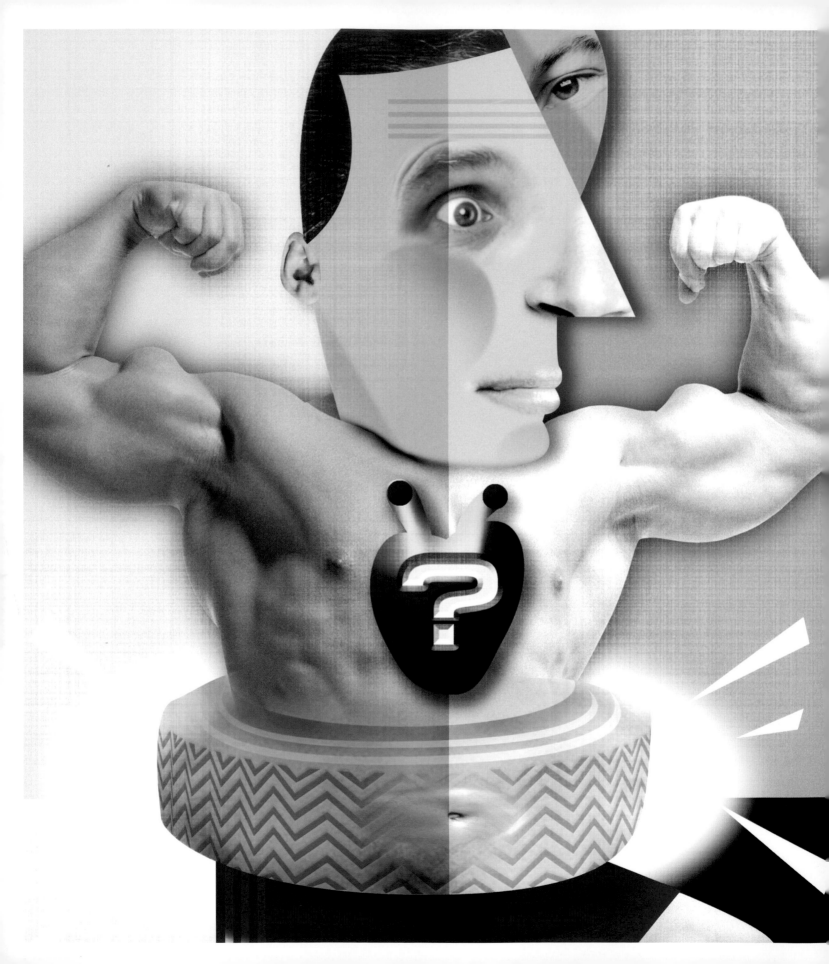

Great Abs in Five Weeks

WANT A MODEL MIDSECTION? IT'S TIME TO STOP DREAMING AND START DOING

Here's your starting point if you've lost your love for your love handles, are apprehensive about taking your shirt off at the beach, or you suck in your gut every time you look in the mirror. This five-week program is your guide to finally dropping the fat and creating the body you've always wanted.

[ITS THREE COMPONENTS INCLUDE]

Ab Workout

Three times per week, you'll do the workout listed, which should take 10–15 minutes. Each week you graduate to a slightly more difficult routine. In each workout, you do the lower-abdominal exercise first, then move to an oblique exercise, and finally to an upper-abdominal move. As you progress, some of the exercises will hit more than one area of the abs.

Since each workout is designed to be a bit more challenging than the previous week's, you'll gain strength and enhance your fitness over the course of the five weeks. Take at least 48 hours rest between workouts before hitting your abs again. If the movements in the five-week program are too difficult, repeat the previous week's exercises, striving to do more reps in each successive workout to build strength. Go to the next week's exercises as soon as you feel you've gained sufficient strength, when you can complete about 12 reps with good form. If the movements are too easy, go to the next week's exercises. If those are still too easy, you can substitute advanced variations from the chapter that covers ab exercises.

Add this program to your current resistance-training program if you currently have one. Though it's not critical, weight training is a good idea because it helps burn calories, increases lean muscle tissue and will help you reach your goals much faster.

Cardio Workout

Starting on page 32, we provide a variety of cardio workouts that you should perform 3–4 times a week to speed up fat loss. Do these concurrently with your ab training. The cardio workouts can be done indoors or out, and increase in duration and intensity over the course of the five weeks so that you're improving your fitness level while increasing fat loss.

Diet

On page 36, we present a five-week diet that builds on itself so you can easily make the transition to eating healthier, low-fat foods. We also offer food choices for your meals to help you get your diet in gear, fuel your metabolism and help peel away the layers of bodyfat in a gradual, almost painless fashion.

The ab exercises strengthen and tone the midsection, while the cardio and diet help burn away bodyfat. Skip one component and you may still see some results, but optimal progress can come only from consistency in all three areas. The choice is yours!

[WEEK 1 WORKOUT]

Do this workout three times during week 1 on nonconsecutive days. Do as many reps as you can with good form; if you can do more than the target number, choose a more difficult movement for that area of the abs (upper, lower or obliques) from next week's workout. Strive to do more reps each workout as you get stronger.

THE ROUTINE

EXERCISE	SETS	REPS
Pelvic Tilt	3	12, 12, 12
Twist	3	15, 15, 15
Curl-Up	3	12, 12, 12

Curl-Up/Upper

[START]

Lie on your back with your feet flat on the floor and knees bent about 60 degrees. Position your arms next to your hips, palms down; your head should be neutrally aligned.

[MOVEMENT]

Curl your torso up, moving your hands toward your feet as your shoulders lift off the floor. Concentrate on feeling your abs contract. Slowly return to the start position.

QUICK TIP
If keeping your hands close to the floor is too difficult, rest your hands on the floor. To increase the difficulty, cross your hands over your chest or clasp them lightly behind your head.

A

B

Pelvic Tilt/Lower

[START]

Lie on your back with your hands out to your sides, legs bent and feet flat on the floor.

[MOVEMENT]

Slowly flatten out your lower back, pressing the small of your back into the floor, then roll your hips toward your chest. Hold for five seconds. Return to the starting position and repeat.

QUICK TIP
The range of motion is extremely small — just go far enough to feel your abs contract and then hold.

A

B

Twist/Obliques

[START]

Sit on the floor with your legs extended and spread in front of you. Place each hand on the same-side shoulder.

[MOVEMENT]

Twist from side to side using deliberately slow movements to prevent momentum, which causes you to cheat. Concentrate on twisting at the waist, not the hips or legs.

QUICK TIP
You can also do this exercise standing, but the seated version helps eliminate lower-body movement.

A

B

[WEEK 1]

[WEEK 2 WORKOUT]

Do this workout three times during week 2 on nonconsecutive days. If you can do more reps with good form than listed, choose more difficult exercises for that target area from next week's program. If you can't do six reps, choose easier exercises from the week 1 workout.

THE ROUTINE

EXERCISE	SETS	REPS
Seated Knee-Up	3	12, 12, 12
Oblique Crunch	3	12, 12, 12
Thigh-Slide Crunch	3	15, 15, 15

Thigh-Slide Crunch/Upper

[START]

Lie on the floor with your knees bent about 60 degrees, feet flat on the floor about shoulder-width apart, palms on your upper thighs.

[MOVEMENT]

Contract your abs and slide your hands toward your knees while lifting your shoulder blades off the floor. Hold briefly and slowly return to the start position.

A

QUICK TIP
Reach toward your knees as high as you can without using momentum; use only your abdominal strength.

B

Oblique Crunch/Obliques

[START]

Lie on your left side, legs on top of each other with your knees bent to reduce the stress on your lower back. Loosely cup your head with your right hand.

[MOVEMENT]

Crunch up as high as you can, keeping the movement in the lateral plane as much as possible to emphasize the obliques. Do both sides.

QUICK TIP
Slightly raise your legs simultaneously as you crunch your upper body to get a better contraction.

Seated Knee-Up/Lower

[START]

Sit at the end of a flat bench (or similar object), legs and feet together, hands grasping the sides of the bench behind your hips.

QUICK TIP
Raising your feet increases the level of difficulty. If necessary, this move can be done on a floor mat.

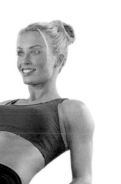

A

[MOVEMENT]

Stabilize your body, lean back slightly and extend your legs down and out in front of you. Contract your abs to bring your knees toward your chest as you simultaneously crunch forward. Keep the motion slow and controlled.

B

[WEEK 2]

[WEEK 3 WORKOUT]

Do this workout three times during week 3 on nonconsecutive days.

THE ROUTINE

EXERCISE	SETS	REPS
Reverse Crunch	3	15, 12, 12
Side Jackknife	2	15, 15, 15
Crossover Crunch	2	12, 12, 12
Crunch (hands on chest)	3	15, 12, 12

Crossover Crunch/Combo

[START]
Lie on your back, right foot on the floor and the left foot crossed over your right knee.

QUICK TIP
To make it less difficult, keep your nonworking elbow against the floor for leverage (as shown).

A

B

[MOVEMENT]
Crunch up to bring your right shoulder blade off the floor, aiming your right shoulder toward your elevated knee. Avoid flapping your elbow. Do both sides.

Side Jackknife/Obliques

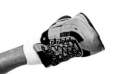

A

B

[START]
Lie on your right side, keeping your left leg over your right one and bending your knees slightly. Place your right hand in a comfortable position; clasp your left hand behind your head.

[MOVEMENT]
Bring your torso and left leg toward each other as you pull with your obliques. Hold the contraction briefly and lower slowly. Do both sides.

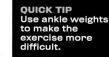

QUICK TIP
Use ankle weights to make the exercise more difficult.

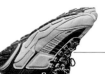

Reverse Crunch/Lower

[START]

Lie faceup on the floor with your hands by your sides, feet up and thighs perpendicular to the floor.

QUICK TIP
To make the exercise more difficult, try it on an incline board or use ankle weights.

[MOVEMENT]

Use your lower abs to roll your pelvis upward to raise your hips off the floor. Your knees will be over your chest. Return under control.

A

B

Crunch (Hands on Chest)/Upper

[START]

Lie faceup on the floor, knees bent and feet flat, hands crossed over your chest.

[MOVEMENT]

As you contract your abs to curl your shoulder blades off the floor, imagine that you're trying to touch your ribcage to your hips as you press your low back into the floor. The range of motion is quite short.

A

B

QUICK TIP
Keep your shoulders off the floor between reps to best stimulate your abs.

[WEEK 3]

[WEEK 4 WORKOUT]

Do this workout three times during week 4 on nonconsecutive days.

Butterfly Crunch/Upper

THE ROUTINE		
EXERCISE	**SETS**	**REPS**
Bent-Knee Hip Raise	3	12, 12, 12
Cross-Body Crunch	2	12, 12, 12
Butterfly Crunch	3	15, 15, 15
Reach & Catch	2	12, 12, 12

A

B

[MOVEMENT]

Curl forward to bring your shoulder blades up, pressing your lower back into the floor. The range of motion is very small.

[START]

Lie faceup with your knees relaxed out to the sides, heels together on the floor.

QUICK TIP
Don't pull on your head in an effort to go higher, and don't press your chin into your chest — keep a space about the size of a small apple between your chin and chest.

Reach & Catch/Combo

A

[MOVEMENT]

Curl your torso as high as you can by contracting your abs, extending both hands to the outside of one knee as if to catch a touchdown pass. Alternate sides or do all your reps for one side first, then the other.

[START]

Lie on your back with your knees bent; place your feet about 2 feet apart on the floor.

QUICK TIP
Really extend as if to make a catch to more effectively work your abs.

B

Bent-Knee Hip Raise & Lower

[START]

This is the same movement as the reverse crunch but with a longer range of motion. Begin with your hands outstretched to your sides, knees bent 60 degrees and your feet just off the floor.

A

QUICK TIP
Straighten your legs to make the movement more difficult.

[MOVEMENT]

Use your lower abs to roll your pelvis upward to raise your hips off the floor. Your knees will be over your chest. Hold briefly at the top and return slowly.

B

Cross-Body Crunch/Combo

[START]

Lie on your back with your knees bent about 60 degrees and your feet flat on the floor. Place one or both hands loosely behind your head.

[MOVEMENT]

Curl up, bringing your right elbow and shoulder across your body, simultaneously bringing your left knee in toward your right elbow. Reach with your elbow as if trying to touch the outside of your knee. Do all reps to one side first, then the other.

A

QUICK TIP
Try not to flap your elbow; make a real effort to bring your shoulder up and toward the opposite knee.

B

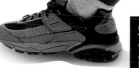

[WEEK 4]

[WEEK 5 WORKOUT]

Do this workout three times during week 5 on nonconsecutive days.

THE ROUTINE

EXERCISE	SETS	REPS
Hip Thrust	3	15, 12, 12
Air Bike	3	12, 12, 12
Straight-Leg Crunch	3	12, 12, 12
Crunch (hands behind head)	3	15, 12, 12

Crunch (Hands Behind Head)/Upper

A

[START]

Lie on your back with your hands loosely cupping your head and feet flat on the floor, knees bent about 60 degrees.

QUICK TIP
The movement is very small, 2–3 inches at most. Avoid letting your shoulder blades touch down as you return to the start.

[MOVEMENT]

Curl up as high as possible without lifting your low back off the floor. Imagine that you're trying to bring your ribcage toward your hips as you push your lower back into the floor.

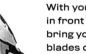

Straight-Leg Crunch/Combo

[START]

Lie on the floor with your legs straight up in the air, which requires your lower abs to work isometrically.

QUICK TIP
To make the exercise easier, slide your glutes up against a wall to support your legs.

[MOVEMENT]

With your arms extended in front of you, curl up to bring your shoulder blades off the floor, reaching toward your toes, then slowly lower back to the start. Don't jerk your body or use momentum; keep it smooth and controlled.

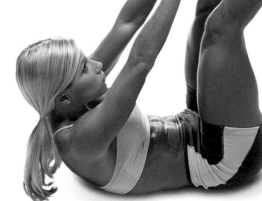

A

B

Hip Thrust Lower

[START]

Lie on the floor with your arms at your sides, palms down. Lift your legs perpendicular to the floor.

[MOVEMENT]

Use your abs to lift your hips only a few inches straight off the floor, pushing your heels toward the ceiling. The range of motion is very small; keep the movement slow and controlled.

QUICK TIP
Try it on an incline board to increase the level of difficulty.

A

B

Air Bike/Combo

QUICK TIP
Don't just flap your elbow across your body; actually rotate your shoulder across.

[START]

Lie on your back with your hands lightly supporting your head. Raise your legs so your thighs are perpendicular and your lower legs are just above parallel to the floor.

[MOVEMENT]

As you curl up, bring your left elbow across your body while drawing your right knee in to meet it, as if riding a bike. Alternate sides, continuing the motion back and forth.

[WEEK 5]

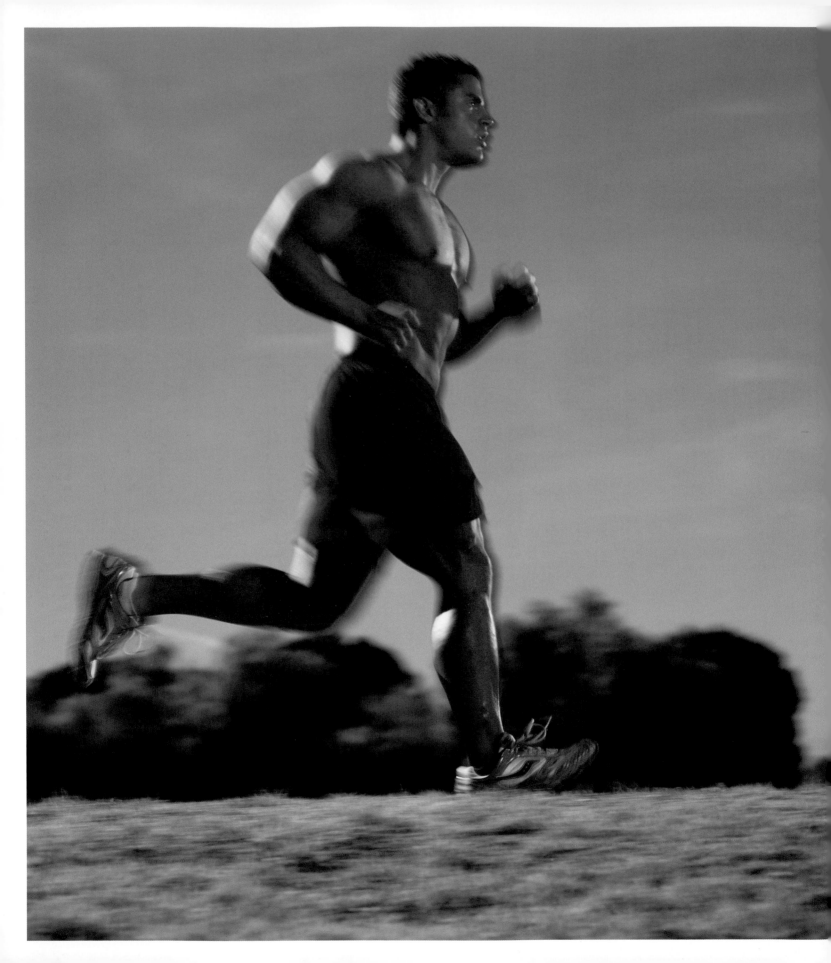

Five-Week Cardio Plan

SPEED UP YOUR FAT LOSS TO REVEAL THE ABS OF YOUR DREAMS

In combination with the five-week ab-training program we've just outlined, you'll also want to add cardiovascular training to your routine. Now, we're not going to ask you to run a marathon or spend hours toiling away on a treadmill. That's fine for advanced athletes, but for the rest of us who have lives outside the gym, it's just not practical or necessary. ❡ Honestly, if you haven't trained much in the past, you'll be surprised at how much benefit you can get from short and sweet cardio workouts. While weight training is the best way to

change your body composition and shape your body over the long haul, one of the best ways to burn fat is through cardiovascular (also called aerobic) exercise. Done properly — that is, keeping your heart rate fairly high for extended periods — aerobic activity is essential for that ultra-lean look.

Besides fat-burning, it's worth noting that cardio activity does a number of other things in the body, including improving your overall fitness and heart health by decreasing risk for diseases such as obesity, hypertension, diabetes and elevated LDL-cholesterol; improving mood and reducing stress; as well as positively affecting a number of other factors linked to overall health. For our purposes, cardio's effect on bodyfat utilization is paramount to helping you realize a well-defined midsection.

The essential elements of your aerobics component include:

■ Warm-up and cool-down
■ The activity you choose
■ How often you do it weekly
■ How long you do it each session
■ The intensity of the exercise session
■ Making progress over the course of the five weeks.

Warm-up and cool-down: Before starting any activity, you need to warm up your working muscles and connective tissue, heart and lungs for 5–10 minutes, both to help prevent injuries and to allow you to work at a high degree of intensity later on. Start off at a very low intensity and gradually work harder until you're breathing more deeply and you break a sweat. Activities that incorporate the body's larger muscle groups, namely the legs, are good choices, including the bicycle, treadmill, stair-stepper and elliptical trainer, or simply do some light calisthenics for a few minutes.

If you want to stretch particular muscles, do so after your warm-up (remember, a warm muscle is more easily stretched than a cold one). After your workout session, light stretching serves as a good cool-down in combination with low-level aerobic activity. The cool-down allows your working muscles and

When it comes to the type of activity you employ for your cardio sessions, you can follow the program exactly, swap the listed activity for something below, or come up with your own alternatives. Don't do the same thing over and over, however, and be aware that some activities may make it difficult to maintain your target heart rate or PE for an extended period. For example, keeping your heart rate steady while cycling outdoors may be a challenge, depending on the route you take.

INDOOR ACTIVITY	OUTDOOR ALTERNATIVE
Treadmill walk	Walk
Treadmill jog	Jog
Treadmill incline walk	Walk hills
Stationary cycle	Cycle
Studio cycle	Climb stadium stairs
Stair-stepper	Inline skate
Versa Climber	Swim
Elliptical trainer	Walk, jog, cycle

Cardio

DAY	MODE	DURATION (MINUTES)*	INTENSITY (% OF MAX HR)	INTENSITY (PE)
1	Stationary bike	20	60%	6
2				
3	Outdoor walk	20	60%	6
4				
5	Elliptical trainer	20	65%	6.5
6				
7				
8	Treadmill	20	65%	6.5
9				
10	Outdoor bike	25	60%–70%	6–7
11				
12	Stair-stepper	25	65%	6.5
13				
14	Elliptical trainer	25	65%	6.5
15				
16	Outdoor jog	25	65%	6.5
17				
18	Stationary bike	30	60%	6
19				
20	Treadmill	30	65%	6.5
21	Stair-stepper	30	70%	7
22				
23	Outdoor jog	35	70%	7
24				
25	Elliptical trainer	30	75%	7.5
26				
27	Outdoor bike	35	70%	7
28	Treadmill	35	65%	6.5
29				
30	Stair-stepper	30	75%	7.5
31				
32	Stationary bike	35	70%	7
33	Elliptical trainer	40	65%	6.5
34				
35	Outdoor run	35	75%	7.5

*Excludes warm-up and cool-down

35-Day Cardio Plan

This progressive five-week cardio program literally leaves nothing to chance. Intensity, duration and frequency are mapped out day by day, and although activities are suggested, you ultimately choose. You can do cardio on the same days as your ab training or regular weight workout — just be sure to do the weights first if you're completing both during the same workout. Or, you can split them apart, doing cardio in the morning and weights at night, for instance.

This program is meant for someone who either hasn't exercised regularly at all in the past or has worked out only sporadically. It's meant to be done in combination with the five-week ab training program on pages 22–31. If the intensity level is too low or you can handle the duration, adjust those variables upward to meet your ability, but stay within your personal limits. Make sure, however, that over the course of the five weeks, you aim to make gains in your cardiovascular condition by increasing the intensity and/or duration and/or frequency over time. Continually challenging yourself as you keep improving is the key to reducing bodyfat while improving your fitness levels.

When scheduling your cardio time, there are a few tricks you can try to speed up the fat-burning process. For instance, some trainees have found success doing cardio first thing in the morning on an empty stomach. Your body may be more apt to burn fat because you don't have as much glycogen in your muscles at this time.

The watchword for taking off that extra layer of fat is consistency. Stick with it, even if the first week or two are tough; by the third week, you'll start to form a habit. Putting all the pieces together isn't easy. Even if you get slightly off track, don't be hard on yourself — just get back in the game. In the end, success or failure is up to you!

circulatory system time to return to normal levels; dropping the heart rate too quickly can cause dizziness and even fainting.

Choose an activity: The type of exercise you choose comes down to what you're capable of doing, what you like doing, equipment available, time constraints and personal goals. Activities that are aerobic are ones that use the large muscle groups, are rhythmic and cardiorespiratory in nature, and can be maintained over a continuous period. Hence, riding a bike for 20 minutes would be considered an aerobic activity; playing chess for 40 minutes would not. Many of the activities you chose from for warming up can also be done as your main activity, as can many group fitness classes. One critical reminder: Choose activities you enjoy doing, because you're much more likely to keep it up than if you do an activity you dislike.

For this five-week session, we mix up the cardio activities, which not only prevent boredom, but also helps keep your body from adapting too quickly to what you're doing. Regularly changing your cardio routine is the best way to keep your body responding to your efforts — that's why this plan changes your aerobic workouts continuously.

Keeping Track of the Details

Frequency of sessions: This refers to the number of workouts you complete per week. The American College of Sports Medicine recommends 3–5 days per week for most aerobic programs. Take no more than two days off between sessions.

How long you should go: Exclusive of the warm-up and cool-down, the exercise duration can vary from as few as five minutes to up to 60 minutes or more. In general, beginners should aim for 10–20 minutes of aerobic work, while individuals with average fitness levels can go 15–45 minutes. Highly fit people can go for 30–60 minutes.

How intensely you should train: Exercise physiologists measure cardio training intensity with what's called age-related maximum heart rate (MHR). Though MHR is an approximation, you can calculate it by subtracting your age from the number 220. An individual who's 30, then, has an MHR of 190. That's an estimate of the maximum number of times a 30-year-old's heart can possibly beat in one minute if it were pumping all-out (obviously, it's not safe to train *that* hard). Use either a heart-rate monitor or actually take your pulse for 10 seconds and multiply by 6 to compute your heart rate in beats per minute. You can then raise or lower your intensity by going faster or slower to train in a certain zone (called target heart-rate training, or THR). This is done by multiplying the relevant percentage (about 60% for beginners to 85% for advanced) by

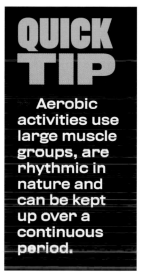

QUICK TIP

Aerobic activities use large muscle groups, are rhythmic in nature and can be kept up over a continuous period.

your MHR. So the 30-year-old who wants to train at 60% of his MHR would want his heart to beat at 114 beats per minute (0.6 x 190), his THR, during his cardio workout.

However, stopping your workout every couple of minutes is difficult at best. If you don't have the benefit of using a heart-rate monitor, you can substitute perceived exertion (PE) for target heart rate to gauge the intensity of your cardio workouts. On a scale of 1–10, with 10 representing the highest level of intensity you can imagine, determine how hard you're working by how you feel. Conveniently, your heart rate and the PE numbers correlate fairly closely, so if you're working at about a 6 on the PE scale, you're most likely working at about 60% of your maximum heart rate. On the five-week program, you'll see both a recommended percentage of your MHR you should be working at (after your warm-up) and the corresponding perceived exertion.

Most people are fairly accurate at pegging the various levels of intensity at which they're working. If you're new to exercise, however, you won't be as adept at judging your PE, but you'll get better with time. Just be honest with yourself when assessing your workload and realize there will be times — when you're tired, if you missed a meal, after your weight workout — when you'll feel like you're working hard no matter what you do. Those are the days when it's better to rest or at least take it easy on yourself in your training.

Ultimately, as your fitness levels improve, you'll be able to train more intensely, but that still doesn't mean you'll want to go all-out. Very high levels of intensity utilize stored sugar (called glycogen) more than bodyfat, which is what we're aiming to burn here. The processes that burn fat require oxygen, so if you're going too fast and can't catch your breath, you're probably burning more stored sugar than fat. Slow down a bit, or alternate high- and low-intensity intervals (explained in a later chapter) to maximize fat-burning.

Your Personal Progression Plan

Making progress: To succeed, a program must continually challenge you as your fitness levels improve. This means making gradual progressions in the frequency, duration and intensity of exercise — but not increasing all the factors at once. You may start doing three 20-minute sessions your first week, but by week five you'll be doing 4–5 sessions for 30 minutes apiece at a higher intensity level. The plan should also be modified for your personal rate of progression. Not everyone adjusts at the same rate, and this depends on many factors, including your age, health status, fitness level, genetics, motivation and more.

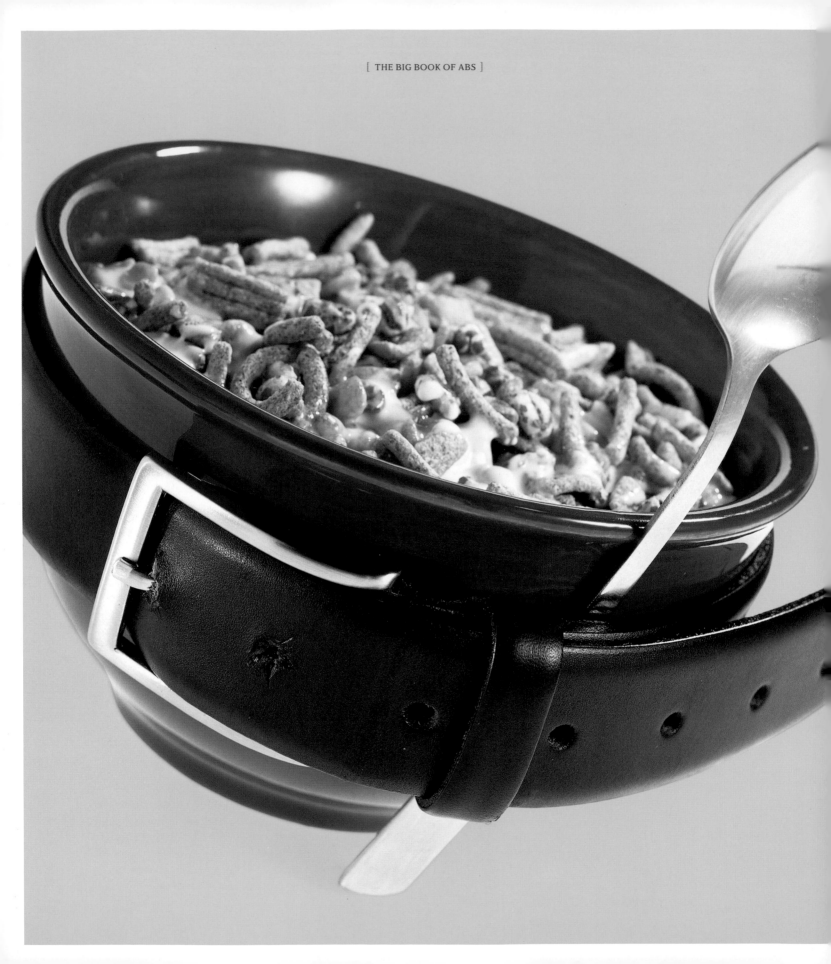

Get Lean in Five Weeks

MAKE EATING RIGHT A REGULAR HABIT WITH THIS 35-DAY PHASE-IN PLAN

Along with exercise and cardio, the third part of the abs equation is your diet. To reach your goal of a well-defined midsection, you must follow a get-lean nutrition plan. Why? Even if you work out hard for an hour every day doing weights in addition to your ab workout, that still leaves 23 more hours for you to wreck all your hard work. Diet is a huge part of the fat-loss equation. It's the backbone of your entire plan, the foundation of a hard body.

But "diet" doesn't mean you can't eat. Your body needs fuel, and that fuel comes in the form of healthy food. The difference is that these guidelines provide the proper fuel for getting lean.

Bodybuilding nutrition consultant Jim Juge says nutrition determines your success or failure, plain and simple. "The diet is 65% of what you need to get in shape," he says. In other words, eating right will produce better results more quickly.

You've got 35 days to reach your goal of shedding as much fat as possible. Go to the grocery store and stock up on the right foods, and throw away those tempting foods that'll derail your progress. Once you make it to the five-week mark, you'll have already changed your eating habits and will find it much easier to continue eating a lean, healthy diet as a lifelong habit.

This five-week plan eases you into a diet that's likely stricter than the one you currently follow. It's one that you should follow the rest of your life, so moderation and balance are essential. The plan progresses in steps, small increments that'll gradually add up to huge triumphs. Follow the guidelines listed for each week, and continue with the previous week's recommendations as the weeks pass. In week 3 you'll still be doing what you learned in weeks 1–2, and so on. By week 5 you'll have developed an essential base of sports-nutrition habits.

The phase-in plan can help you reduce bodyfat while maintaining your lean muscle tissue. By making small adjustments in your food choices and caloric intake that help maximize fat-burning, staying on your diet is far easier. Other diets may be more restrictive, but that doesn't mean they'll lead to greater success at shedding bodyfat. "There's a point of negative return for anyone trying to shed bodyfat," says Bonnie Modugno, RD, of Santa Monica, California. "Conventional wisdom seems to indicate that any more than a 10%–15% decrease in caloric intake will not help you lose bodyfat more quickly." She explains that while you can indeed lose more weight by further restricting calories, much of that will be water and lean muscle tissue, which the body turns to when it senses drastic calorie reductions.

Neither is this a crash diet on which you'll lose a lot of pounds quickly. "A reasonable expectation is that you can lose a half-pound to a pound of bodyfat per week," notes Modugno. Factors like metabolic rate and the amount of muscle mass you hold onto can also accelerate how much bodyfat you burn.

Your Get-Lean Principles
[WEEK 1] ASSESS YOURSELF

Starting on the first day of the week, keep a food journal for three full days. Include the times you eat, what you eat, how much you eat and how hungry you are when you eat it. If you have half a bag of Doritos after dinner, make sure you write it down.

Take note of how your schedule affects your diet. What times do you have available to eat during the day? What times are too hectic to even think about getting food? When do you get hungry? In addition, take a few photos of yourself to keep your motivation up. Focus on your goal, whether it's a reunion, vacation or special occasion, so you'll have something to strive for. Take front, side and back pictures and post the photos on your fridge at home. Keep looking at those photos and envision how much fitter you'll look and feel in a few weeks.

Day 4: Now, harness all of that information and write down three goals for yourself. Is there a bad habit you'd like to break? Do you go eight hours without eating? Is there a single fresh vegetable in that three-day food diary?

You're not going to completely make over your diet overnight, nor would you want to. Your chance of success is infinitely better if you set some reasonable, realistic, attainable goals rather than vowing to subsist entirely on scrambled egg whites, grilled chicken breasts and steamed broccoli.

Day 5: Write a list of your pros and cons about eating a healthier diet. Be completely honest! Are finances a barrier? Time? Do you associate dieting with a loss of a social life? For the next couple of days, think about how you might overcome those "cons" when they inevitably arise. Write at least one countering technique you can use for each.

[WEEK 2] EAT MORE FREQUENTLY + UP YOUR PROTEIN INTAKE

Instead of thinking "breakfast, lunch and dinner," start thinking of those same meals spread over 4–5 meals. Going 5–7 hours between meals makes you less likely to lose fat, more likely to store fat and more likely to overeat when you're hungry. Your smaller, more frequent meals should range between about 400 and 700 calories, but don't get hung up on calories just yet. For now, just get in the habit of eating every 3–4 hours.

Things to Bring: It's easier to stick to an eating schedule if you're prepared. Stock up on a few of these items for time-crunched situations that don't allow you to prepare a meal.

- Pop-top or single-serve pouches of water-packed tuna
- Turkey or beef jerky (watch the salt)
- Instant packets of oatmeal (just add water or fat-free milk)
- Protein bars and shake packets
- Fresh fruit, baby carrots, etc.
- Light popcorn
- Yogurt or mini-containers of cottage cheese
- Hard-boiled eggs (boil a dozen, then refrigerate)
- Any kind of nuts (except macadamia)

In addition, eat at least 1 gram of protein per pound of bodyweight daily. If your protein intake is too low on a restricted-calorie diet, you'll start losing muscle tissue in addition to any fat you're lucky enough to shed. A high protein intake will help you preserve lean mass during your dieting phase. An individual who weighs 175 pounds and is eating five meals a day would want to get about 35 grams of protein at each meal.

QUICKTIP Choose lean, high-quality proteins like egg whites, poultry, lean red meat and protein supplements. Many cuts of red meat are typically very high in saturated fat, so choose the leanest cuts available. Cuts of "round" and "loin" are usually your best bets.

QUICKTIP If you eat a lot of fast food, make an effort to consume healthier meals. For instance, try grilled chicken breast sandwiches instead of deep-fried chicken patties or hamburgers. Eat a side salad with a low-fat dressing instead of french fries.

[WEEK 3] WATCH YOUR CARBS + CHANGE YOUR PORTIONS

Keeping an eye on your carbohydrate intake is one proven way to help you lose weight. Besides switching to complex carbs that are as unprocessed as possible, cut back on them significantly on days when your activity level is low or you're not working out.

This ensures that your energy will be high and that you're not overconsuming carbs, which can then be stored as fat.

The easiest guide we can give you is to choose carbs that are closest to their original form. Here are some examples:

ORIGINAL SOURCE	GOOD SOURCE	ADEQUATE SOURCE	PROCESSED
Wheat	Whole-wheat bread/pita/ bagel/cracker/ pasta	White bread, regular pasta, Saltine cracker, water bagel	Croutons, boxed macaroni 'n' cheese, bagel chips, cheese-flavored crackers
Potato	Baked potato, low-fat potato salad, low-fat mashed potatoes with skin	Air-baked french fries	Boxed instant mashed potatoes, potato chips
Rice	Brown rice	White rice	Rice Krispies
Oats	Old-fashioned oatmeal	Instant packet oatmeal	Oatmeal cookie
Apple	No-sugar-added natural applesauce, dried apples	Apple juice	Apple butter

Start eating more toward the left of the chart and less toward the right. Chances are you'll get less added sugar and fewer preservatives, fewer calories and less saturated fat, less sodium and more fiber and water. You may even be surprised at how tasty the foods are. Also, reduce simple sugars as much as possible, including sweets, sodas, pastries and cakes. It's far healthier to eat complex carbs rather than simple carbs, with the exception of fresh fruit.

If fat loss is your goal, you also need to reduce calories to some extent so your total calorie intake is less than your total calorie expenditure. Portion size is the simplest method of weight control and much easier than counting calories. Stick with portions that fit in your palm, visualized as follows:
- One serving meat or fish = deck of cards
- One serving rice or pasta = tight fist
- One baked potato = computer mouse
- One serving of cheese – four dice
- One serving of butter, mayonnaise or other fats = thumb tip.
If you count calories, base your daily intake on the following:
- For fat loss: Your weight x 12
- For maintenance: Your weight x 15
- For mass gain: Your weight x 18.

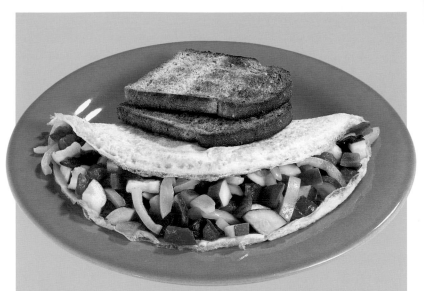

Breakfast

 BOWL OF HIGH-FIBER CEREAL WITH 1 CUP OF FAT-FREE MILK. Choose a cereal that has more than 5 grams of fiber per serving, such as Kashi Good Friends, Kashi Go Lean, bran flakes or shredded wheat. Sorry, Count Chocula doesn't make the cut.
330 calories, 68 g carbs, 11 g protein, 1.5 g fat

 WHOLE-GRAIN ENGLISH MUFFIN WITH TOMATO SLICES AND TWO PIECES OF MELTED LOW-FAT CHEESE. For muffins, try Matthews or Thomas'. For the cheese, try a fresh Jarlsberg/muenster light or Alpine Lace.
280 calories, 46 g carbs, 16 g protein, 4 g fat

 FIVE EGG-WHITE VEGETABLE OMELET (ONION, TOMATO AND BELL PEPPER). You can use one whole egg plus four egg whites, or a small container of egg substitute. Use nonstick cooking spray to fry them in a pan. Add two slices of dry whole-wheat toast or a dry whole-grain english muffin.
300 calories, 47 g carbs, 25 g protein, 3 g fat

 ONE CUP OF LOW-FAT OR FAT-FREE COTTAGE CHEESE WITH TWO TABLESPOONS OF CRUNCHY CEREAL, WHEAT GERM OR GROUND FLAXSEEDS. You can use your fruit serving as a sweetener for the cottage cheese.
300 calories, 36 g carbs, 30 g protein, 3.5 g fat

 UNSWEETENED OATMEAL OR STEEL OATS. Mix ½ cup of oatmeal with water, fat-free milk or soymilk. Get your fruit serving by adding two tablespoons of raisins or 1 cup of berries.
250 calories, 45 g carbs, 11 g protein, 3 g fat

 PROTEIN SHAKE. In a blender, mix one 100-calorie scoop of protein powder (any brand will do) with 1 cup of fat-free milk, half a banana, 1 cup of berries and ice cubes.
340 calories, 60 g carbs, 32 g protein, 1.5 g fat

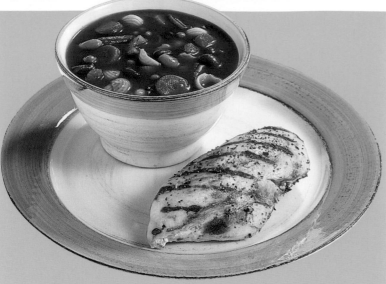

Lunch

 SOUP AND CHICKEN OR FISH. A bowl of any noncreamy, vegetable-based soup, such as minestrone, vegetable barley or tomato, with 6 ounces of grilled, skinless chicken breast or fish. 500 calories, 58 g carbs, 54 g protein, 6 g fat

 SANDWICH AND SALAD. 4 ounces of lean turkey breast, grilled chicken breast, lean ham or tuna salad on two slices of whole-grain or oat-bran bread or a pita. Use mustard, ketchup, barbecue sauce or low-fat mayo for flavor. Add a side salad with 2 tablespoons of low-fat dressing or 1 tablespoon of vinaigrette dressing. 500 calories, 57 g carbs, 43 g protein, 12 g fat

LARGE SALAD AND A SLICE OF WHOLE-GRAIN BREAD. Top the greens with 4 ounces of lean protein, such as plain tuna, grilled salmon, shrimp, skinless chicken breast or turkey breast. Add ½ cup of chickpeas, beans or corn. Flavor with 2-4 tablespoons of low-fat dressing. 500 calories, 65 g carbs, 46 g protein, 8 g fat

 FIVE EGG-WHITE OMELET, WITH ANY VEGETABLE COMBINATION, AND TWO SLICES OF WHOLE-WHEAT TOAST. Add a slice of low-fat cheese and a fresh fruit salad on the side. 500 calories, 80 g carbs, 37 g protein, 7 g fat

 PLAIN HAMBURGER, TURKEY BURGER OR VEGGIE BURGER. Have as many sliced tomatoes as you'd like and an orange or a grapefruit on the side, but no bun and no fries. *For a beef burger:* 500 calories, 45 g carbs, 25 g protein, 20 g fat

 BAKED POTATO WITH STEAMED CHOPPED BROCCOLI, ½ CUP OF SHREDDED LOW-FAT CHEESE AND 1 CUP OF VEGETABLE SOUP. When eating out, you can substitute 3 tablespoons of Parmesan cheese if low-fat cheese isn't available. 500 calories, 75 g carbs, 27 g protein, 8 g fat

For example, a 170-pound person who wants to lose weight would eat about 2,000 calories per day. Another method you can use is to keep a three-day diary of your usual food intake (in which you're maintaining your weight) and calculate an average of the three days' total calories. For weight loss, aim to reduce your caloric intake by about 300–500 per day, or eat 150–250 fewer calories daily and burn the balance through cardio activities.

[WEEK 4] LIMIT SATURATED FAT + DRINK LIKE A FISH

While you don't need to cut fat out of your diet completely, some fats are far more desirable than others. Here's a cheat sheet to help get you started.

GOOD-FOR-YOU FAT SOURCES	USE ONLY IN MODERATION
Nuts	Butter
Olive oil	Sour cream
Avocado	Partially hydrogenated oil
Canola oil	Coconut oil
Peanut butter	Whole milk and cheese
Fatty fish	Marbled cuts of beef and poultry with skin

Each dietary fat gram has 9 calories, while each protein and carbohydrate gram has 4 calories. The reason many people watch their fat intake on weight-reducing diets is that it packs so many calories in a small amount of food.

QUICKTIP On packaged foods, make sure you check labels for calories and serving size — some use unusually small serving sizes so they can appear to show a low calorie total.

Also, you want to drink at least a gallon of water per day. This will keep you hydrated and healthy, not to mention full when you might otherwise want to grab a high-calorie snack. Water should be your primary beverage during a weight-loss or get-lean phase, though many dieters rely on diet sodas, Crystal Light and other low-calorie sweetened drinks.

The easiest way to monitor your fluid intake is urine color and volume. The lighter and more of it, the better. If it's dark and concentrated, you need to drink more.

QUICKTIP For optimal performance and recovery, drink 2 cups of water before, during and after exercise.

[WEEK 5] GET LEAN

You'll often hear fitness athletes and bodybuilders use the phrase "eating clean." This means eating foods that are packed with muscle-building nutrients without extras like refined sugar, sodium and trans fats.

QUICKTIP Here's an easy way to clean up your diet without monumental effort or expense: Five days a week, cook one meal from scratch. At that one meal, include at least one serving of vegetables, a lean protein and one serving of a starchy carb. If you can, make extra so you can eat leftovers the next day.

Eating-clean staple foods include:
- Egg whites/eggs
- Lean ground beef/turkey/chicken breast
- Salmon/tuna or other fish
- Potatoes/yams
- Whole-grain bread or pasta, oatmeal
- Low-fat or fat-free milk, cheese, yogurt, cottage cheese
- Fresh and frozen vegetables and fruit
- High-fiber boxed cereals
- To flavor: Mrs. Dash, Molly McButter, cinnamon, nutmeg

QUICKTIP To stay motivated and deal with cravings, schedule a cheat meal on Sunday so you're ready to start the week fully motivated. If you feel deprived during the week, concentrate on the cheat meal to come, knowing you can eat absolutely anything you want to. Remember, though, it's just one cheat meal, not an entire day. Afterward, get right back on the wagon with your next scheduled meal.

[AFTER 5 WEEKS] NOW WHAT?

So you made it through 35 days and you've noticed some changes in the way you feel and the way you look. Where do you go from here? This diet was designed to ease you into long-term healthy eating, so you can continue with this plan indefinitely.

Though you shouldn't expect a drastic weight loss, if you're still not losing weight after five weeks, cut about 250 calories from your day's totals (a small snack). If you're doing cardio, you should be able to achieve about a 500-calorie deficit per day, or 3,500 per week, which equals about a pound. Continue adjusting your calories until you achieve the weight loss you seek.

Snacks

1) ONE PIECE OF FRUIT with two slices of low-fat cheese. 200 calories, 22 g carbs, 8 g protein, 4 g fat
2) A SPORTS BAR with 200 calories or less. 200 calories, 29 g carbs, 14 g protein, 6 g fat
3) BOILED EDAMAME (1½ cups soybeans). 200 calories, 16 g carbs, 18 g protein, 9 g fat
4) WHOLE-WHEAT PITA BREAD with 2 teaspoons of natural peanut butter. 200 calories, 39 g carbs, 9 g protein, 6 g fat
5) ONE SLICED APPLE with 1 tablespoon of natural peanut butter. 200 calories, 25 g carbs, 4 g protein, 8 g fat
6) 8 OUNCES FAT-FREE OR LOW-FAT FLAVORED YOGURT (any variety that is 200 calories or less). 200 calories, 22 g carbs, 12 g protein, 3 g fat

Dinner
ALSO: Any lunches (page 40) with a single serving of fruit.

 CHICKEN STIR-FRY. 6 ounces of boneless, skinless chicken breast and 1 cup of vegetables, stir-fried in 2 teaspoons of vegetable oil and low-sodium soy sauce. Serve with ¾ cup of cooked brown rice or couscous. 550 calories, 41 g carbs, 61 g protein, 16 g fat

 LEAN STEAK, SALAD AND VEGETABLES. Flavor the salad (any size) with 1 tablespoon of vinaigrette dressing. The vegetables you eat with your 6-ounce steak are also up to you: Spinach, broccoli, green beans, asparagus and cauliflower are great choices. 550 calories, 15 g carbs, 50 g protein, 34 g fat

 GRILLED OR BAKED FISH WITH SALAD, STEAMED VEGETABLES AND A PLAIN BAKED SWEET POTATO. For the salad, mix lettuce and tomatoes, then use 2 tablespoons of low-fat dressing. Choose any 6-ounce cut of tuna, halibut, salmon, swordfish or sea bass. 550 calories, 54 g carbs, 61 g protein, 9 g fat

 HAMBURGER, TURKEY BURGER OR VEGGIE BURGER, WITH STEAMED VEGETABLES. Serve on a standard bun or whole-wheat pita bread. Add a mixed green salad with 1 teaspoon of olive oil, adding vinegar and lemon juice to taste. 550 calories, 47 g carbs, 38 g protein, 22 g fat

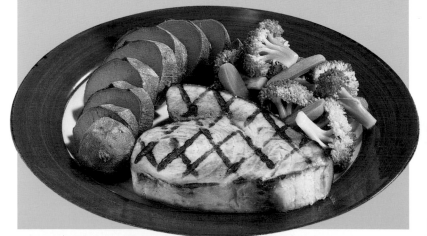

[CHAPTER THREE]

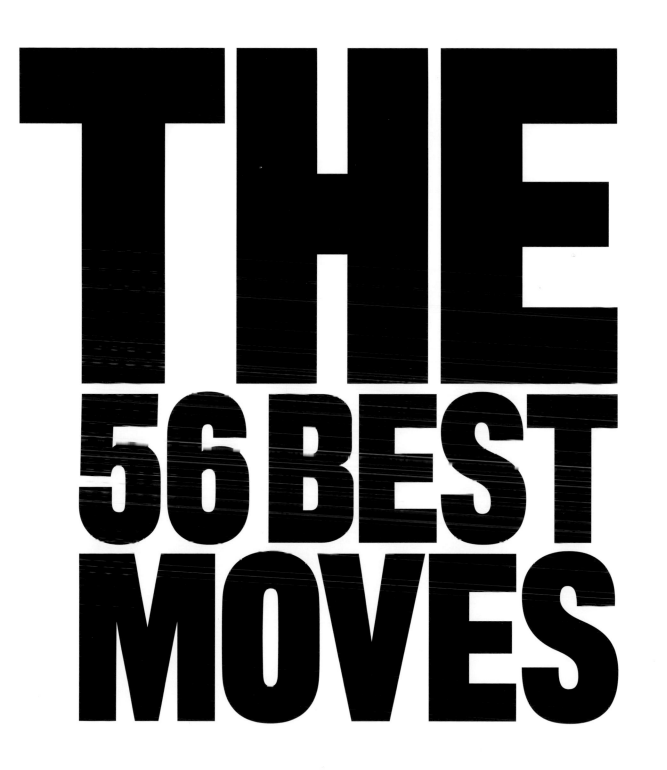

THE 56 BEST MOVES

1) THE BODY'S FOUNDATION

The abdominal muscles serve a purpose far greater than that of making us look good. Coupled with the muscles of the low back, the abs form a natural wall around your entire midsection. When contracted, these muscles increase intra-abdominal pressure and greatly enhance the stability of the spine. Strong abdominal muscles promote good posture and a healthy back.

2) BASIC MOVEMENTS

Proper strength and coordination are required to perform advanced abdominal exercises. Therefore, beginners should start with basic exercises. As your strength and coordination increase, more advanced exercises can be incorporated into your routine. Beginners should also be more concerned about form than reaching rep goals; if you fatigue, take a short break and pick it up from there.

3) CONTROL

As with any exercise, abdominal movements should be performed with strict form in a slow, controlled manner. This will minimize the risk of injury, as some exercises can stress the low back. Slow movements increase the intensity of the contraction and reduce momentum. Momentum is created with fast, swinging motions, which opens the door for injury, not to mention detracting from the overall quality of your workout.

4) RANGE OF MOTION

Usually you want to perform an exercise through its entire range of motion to promote flexibility and maximize muscle-fiber recruitment. Ab training is a little different. In fact, limiting the movement to a fairly short range of motion, as in going to about 30 degrees above the horizontal on floor crunches, will allow complete contraction while minimizing hip-flexor involvement. Movements beyond about 45 degrees, as with full sit-ups, don't result in additional contraction or stimulation of the abs.

5) CONSTANT TENSION

The ab muscles recover extremely fast, so if you rest between reps, even if only for a second, it becomes difficult to adequately fatigue the muscle. To avoid such a breach of form, maintain constant tension on your abdominals by stopping just short of the endpoint during the return phase of the movement.

6) ORDER

Although exercise order is not crucial for ab development, the lower portion of the rectus abdominis is typically the weakest and requires the most coordination to work. In general, work your lower-ab region before the upper abs and obliques, but switch things up on occasion.

7) OBLIQUES

The obliques are called upon during all twisting and rotary movements at the waist. Most upper- and lower-ab exercises can be modified to incorporate the obliques by directing one shoulder toward the opposite knee or by angling a knee toward the opposite shoulder.

8) RESISTANCE

The resistance used in abdominal training typically consists of nothing more than your bodyweight. If your abs are weak or you're just starting a program, consider easier variations; as you progress and your midsection becomes stronger, arm and foot positions can be changed to add difficulty. You can further increase the resistance by adding weight or changing the angle of the exercise. Regardless, the appropriate resistance should be used to elicit the desired number of repetitions.

9) BREATHING

Proper breathing must eventually be learned if it's not instinctively adapted. When exercising your abs, breathe in through your nose during the relaxation phase and forcefully exhale through the mouth at the point of complete contraction. Removing air from the lungs permits a more complete and intense contraction.

10) LOW BACK

Virtually every muscle group has an opposing muscle group that needs to be trained for balance and symmetry (biceps/triceps, hamstrings/quads, etc.). The antagonist muscles to the abdominals are those of the low back. Exercises such as back extensions and deadlifts need to be part of your routine to prevent an imbalance in the muscular development of your core.

Performance Pointers

THE 16 KEYS TO DEVELOPING PERFECT FORM AND REACHING YOUR GOALS

11) CONTRACTION

To get the most out of each exercise, you must focus on feeling the contraction. Beginners often lack the discipline and experience, while seasoned lifters may lose the concentration necessary to feel each rep. Without such focus, form can deteriorate and you simply go through the motions. You may find it helpful to place one hand on your midsection, not only to physically feel the contraction but also as a reminder to concentrate on the movement and to momentarily hold the contraction.

12) UPPER VS. LOWER ABS

Though the rectus abdominis is one muscle, you can emphasize the lower region more strongly by securing your upper body and rotating your hips/pelvis toward your ribcage. Keeping your lower body anchored and curling your upper torso toward your hips works the upper abs more strongly. For all practical purposes, you can't isolate one region or another.

13) A WORD ABOUT REPS

Your goals for the shape of your midsection should dictate how many reps you do. For one thing, the abs have a greater endurance component than most muscle groups, which may explain why they're often trained more frequently with higher repetitions. That said, if you want a strong, well-toned midsection, perform about 20 reps per set with moderate resistance. If your goal is to develop thicker abs with noticeable peaks and valleys, use a traditional regimen of heavy resistance with lower reps. Select an exercise or a resistance that allows you to do 10–12 reps, which is slightly higher than for other bodyparts. In either case, the last few reps should be difficult to complete and cause a burning sensation in the ab muscles.

14) VARIETY

Once you've mastered the basic abdominal exercises and built a solid foundation, add different movements to your ab program. Choosing a variety of exercises serves three purposes: 1) It "shocks" the muscle, preventing it from becoming accustomed to the same exercise; 2) it allows the muscle to be stressed from different angles, maximizing growth by ensuring greater muscle-fiber utilization; and 3) it allows you to choose more difficult moves as you get stronger, allowing you to make further improvements as you progress.

15) SPINAL ALIGNMENT

Although your spine flexes during most abdominal movements (especially those for the upper abs), you should keep your cervical spine (neck), head and shoulders aligned while exercising. Proper positioning will prevent unwanted forces from causing potential injury to the neck. One of the most critical components in achieving and maintaining alignment is hand placement. If you interlock your hands behind your neck, you'll likely pull your head forward and disrupt alignment. Instead, cup your hands behind your ears or place your hands lightly alongside your head to support it.

16) REST PERIODS

After you complete your set, rest to allow your abs to recover so you can complete your next set. If you start too early, they'll still be fatigued and you'll fall short of your goal. In general, beginners should take a little longer between sets, as should individuals who are training for ab strength. If you're advanced or training for muscle endurance, you can keep your rest intervals shorter. You can also add intensity to any workout simply by cutting your usual rest period by several seconds.

Intensity Control

EXERCISE VARIATIONS TO INCREASE/DECREASE DIFFICULTY

Many basic ab exercises can be made easier or more difficult simply by changing the placement of your hands and/or feet. Here are some of the common alterations you can make to most crunch movements that don't involve machines or other equipment.

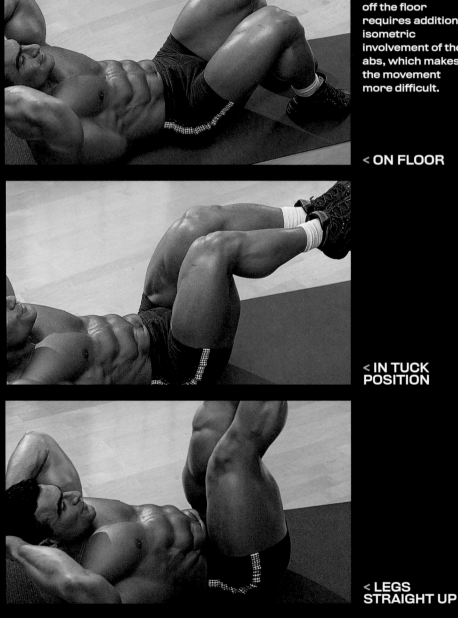

Foot Placement
Raising your feet off the floor requires additional isometric involvement of the abs, which makes the movement more difficult.

< ON FLOOR

< IN TUCK POSITION

< LEGS STRAIGHT UP

LESS DIFFICULT

MORE DIFFICULT

Hand Placement

With your hands close to your center of gravity, the amount of resistance (the weight of your upper body) is reduced, making the movement easier. With your hands farther away from your center of gravity, the exercise becomes more difficult.

Angle of Movement

Ab exercises done on the floor or a flat bench are easier to execute than on a decline bench. Increasing the bench angle further increases the difficulty. The same goes for some reverse-crunch movements done on an incline board.

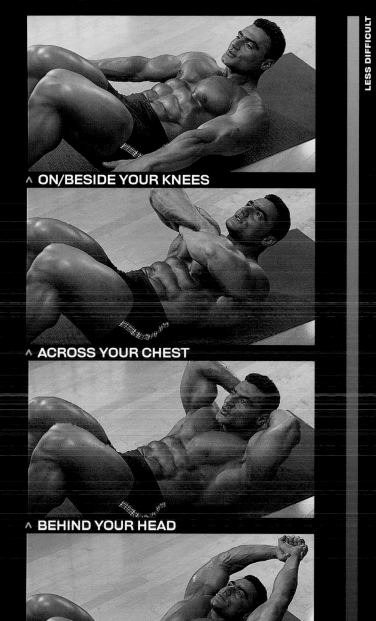

^ ON/BESIDE YOUR KNEES

^ ACROSS YOUR CHEST

^ BEHIND YOUR HEAD

^ EXTENDED OVER YOUR HEAD

LESS DIFFICULT

MORE DIFFICULT

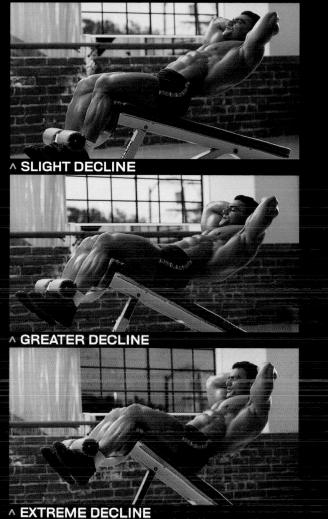

^ SLIGHT DECLINE

^ GREATER DECLINE

^ EXTREME DECLINE

LESS DIFFICULT

MORE DIFFICULT

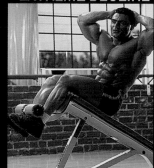

Adding a Twist

Most crunch exercises can be made to include the obliques simply by adding a cross-body movement, bringing one shoulder up and aiming it toward the opposite knee. The key is to point your shoulder and reach — not just flap your elbow. First use forward flexion to bring your torso up, then lead with your shoulder and ribcage, not with your elbow.

Glute-Up

This basic exercise is ideal for those who have little experience training abs directly. Substitute it for lower-ab movements that are too difficult when you first start out.

A

CAUTION
Keep your head in neutral alignment.

FORM
Don't allow your hips to drop to the floor at the bottom.

POSITION
Begin in modified push-up position on your toes with your feet together.

POSITION
Rest your forearms on the floor, your elbows bent about 90 degrees.

B

FORM
At the top, you should be in a high-bridge position.

BREATH
Hold your breath until you reach the top of the rep, then exhale.

MOVEMENT
Push your glutes toward the ceiling. Squeeze your abs tightly to shorten the distance between your hips and ribcage.

SPEED
Use a moderate rate of speed and control the movement at all times.

SKILL
LEVEL

1

[FASTFACT]

You can also perform this move as a warm-up before your other ab exercises. Make sure your motion is smooth and controlled as your muscles warm up.

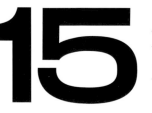

Do three sets of up to **15 reps.** When you can do that comfortably, it's time to choose a more difficult exercise.

[TIP01]

Instead of a flat or arched back, bridge (round) your back slightly in the bottom position; this is safer because it discourages you from arching your back as you weaken.

Leg Lift With Exercise Ball

SETUP
Snugly position
an exercise ball
between your feet
and press them
together to keep
the ball in place.

POSITION
Raise your feet
until you feel
your low back is
flush with the
floor. This is your
start position.

This beginner-level
movement can be done
at home or at the gym.
As you become stronger,
increase the range of
motion or use a heavier
ball to continue making
progress.

MOVEMENT
Raise your legs straight up
6–12 inches in a smooth,
controlled motion.

POSITION
Lie faceup on the floor.
Place your hands
under your glutes.

A

FORM
Keep your legs
straight throughout
the movement.

BREATH
Exhale only
after you
reach the
top position.

MOVEMENT
As you lower the ball,
make sure it doesn't
touch the floor, which
reduces the load on
your abdominals and
the effectiveness of
the exercise.

B

SKILL
LEVEL

[FASTFACT]

Use this move as a warm-up
for a beginning-level workout
or, after your abs are well-
fatigued, finish off your routine
with it to really feel them burn.

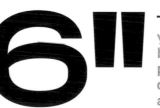

The minimum height
you need to lift the
ball from the starting
position to ensure
contraction of your
abdominals.

[TIP02]

Your low back should be flush
with the floor throughout the
range of motion. If it begins
to lift, adjust your starting
position to begin with your feet
a little higher off the floor.

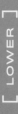

[LOWER]

Leg Raise

You can easily adjust the difficulty of this classic movement by using a lighter or heavier dumbbell.

SPEED
Raise and lower your feet using a controlled motion.

SETUP
Position a light dumbbell between your feet. Squeeze your feet and legs together to hold it in place.

A

FORM
Keep your legs straight throughout the range of motion.

POSITION
Lower your legs no farther than parallel to the floor.

POSITION
Grasp the end of the bench to stabilize your body.

B

MOVEMENT
Use your lower abs to raise your legs until they're perpendicular to the bench.

BREATH
Exhale after you reach the top position.

SKILL
LEVEL

2

[FASTFACT]

Using a slight knee bend decreases the length of the lever your abs pull upward, which makes the movement less difficult.

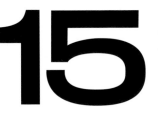

15

Once you can do **15 reps** with good form, use a heavier dumbbell or a more advanced exercise. Do three sets.

[TIP03]

To really burn out your lower abs, after you do as many reps as you can with the weight in place, drop it and continue the set until you can't do any more reps.

LOWER

Exercise-Ball Reverse Crunch

POSITION
Grasp a weighted barbell behind your head for support.

POSITION
Lie on top of the ball, making sure your body is balanced.

Although you perform this exercise like the reverse crunch, it requires additional stabilizers and can be done through a greater range of motion.

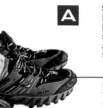

SETUP
Place the exercise ball in front of a sturdy object, like a power rack or Smith machine.

POSITION
Your feet should be off the floor and about even with your glutes.

FORM
Keep your feet together as you complete the movement.

MOVEMENT
Contract your abs to slowly bring your knees toward your chest until your hips reach about a 90-degree angle.

BREATH
Exhale as you reach the point of peak contraction.

MOVEMENT
Lift the lower portion of your glutes off the ball at the top of the movement. Keep your knees bent about 90 degrees.

MAKE IT HARDER
Lock your knees at a larger angle, about 135 degrees. You can also place a light dumbbell between your feet.

[TIP04]
Don't just kick your feet in and out; keep your knees locked at 90 degrees and squeeze your abs.

[FASTFACT]
More advanced trainees can do a bodyweight exercise like hanging knee or leg raises first, then quickly follow up with this move to really hit the lower-ab region.

SKILL LEVEL

2

Glute-Up With Exercise Ball

A

POSITION
Place the ball under your lower thighs and knees.

POSITION
Your feet should be together, legs fully extended. Keep your back flat in the start position.

POSITION
Place your hands on the floor outside shoulder-width apart, arms fully extended.

SETUP
Select a ball size that allows your body to be parallel to the floor in this position.

Tougher than it looks, this exercise works your lower abs and the other stabilizing muscles that make up your core.

FORM
Make sure your legs remain straight and that your feet don't roll off the ball as you descend.

MOVEMENT
Push your glutes toward the ceiling while consciously contracting your abs.

B

FORM
Your hands do not leave this position.

MOVEMENT
The ball should roll down to your shins or toes, depending on how high you can get your glutes in the air.

SKILL LEVEL

2

[FASTFACT]
Try combining this movement with other exercise-ball moves in a single routine to really challenge your abs. That's a smart way to make your muscles work harder.

MAKE IT EASIER
If this movement is too difficult, try it with your feet on the floor. You can also do the toes-on-floor version as the second half of a superset in which you perform the exercise-ball version first.

[TIP05]
This exercise can be performed at home, but make sure you use a smooth surface. Carpeting can cause an uneven resistance that makes the movement awkward.

Partner-Assisted Leg Raise

This move effectively targets your lower-abdominal region. Perform it as your last low-ab exercise and go to failure.

SETUP
Your partner should be ready to quickly catch your feet, then immediately and forcefully push them back down. As you fatigue, he/she should apply slightly less force.

POSITION
Lie faceup on a mat, legs straight (but not locked out) and head aligned with your spine.

SPEED
Fight your partner's push on the negative to fully work your abs in the eccentric contraction.

FORM
Your feet shouldn't touch down at the bottom, which would allow your abs to rest.

POSITION
Your partner should stand with his/her foot on each side of your head. Grasp his/her ankles firmly.

BREATH
Exhale as you reach the top, then quickly inhale and hold your breath as you fight the negative.

MOVEMENT
Contract your abs to bring your feet up directly over your chest.

FORM
Keep your legs and feet together, bringing them up as a single unit.

MOVEMENT
Your glutes should come off the pad just a bit at the top to ensure contraction of your lower abs.

A

B

[FASTFACT]

Your glutes should just barely lift off the mat at the top so that your pelvis rotates. If your glutes aren't coming off the mat, you're not completely contracting your abs.

MAKE IT HARDER

If you find you can handle more than 15 reps, cut your rest periods in half so that your abs aren't fully recovered for your next set. Or try moving as slowly as you can on the negative portion of the rep.

[TIP06]

Fighting the negative works your abs in a way they're probably not used to, so make sure you engage your partner to give you a thorough workout.

SKILL LEVEL

3

[LOWER]

Hanging Run in Place

Do this exercise at the end of your lower-ab routine. The fast pace works your fast-twitch fibers for speed, but you don't get the same degree of resistance as with most other lower-ab moves.

POSITION
Your body should be erect. Don't lean forward as you would for dips.

POSITION
At a vertical bench or dip station, straighten your arms and hang freely. Don't lock out your elbows.

MOVEMENT
Without swinging, bring one knee as high as possible toward your midsection.

[FASTFACT]
This isn't a traditional bodybuilding move, but it develops speed and muscular endurance when you increase the time component. For pure bodybuilding exercises, do hanging knee or leg raises.

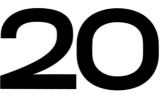

20

Start with a **20-second** set (as opposed to a prescribed number of reps) and work your way up to 60 seconds.

SKILL LEVEL

3

[TIP07]
Your lower abs kick in more the higher you bring your knees. Your objective shouldn't be to do as many reps as possible but to get your knees as high as you possibly can.

FORM
Keep your toes pointed.

GRIP
Grasp the handles just outside shoulder width.

MOVEMENT
Alternate legs, bringing one knee up while you're lowering the opposite knee.

SPEED
Do this movement fairly quickly, as if you're running.

Hanging Knee Raise

This one will really tax you — hanging freely requires greater body control than supported movements.

BREATH
Exhale as you reach the uppermost position.

MOVEMENT
Use your abs to bring your knees as high as you can into your chest.

POSITION
Allow your body to hang freely, arms fully extended.

FORM
Try to get your knees above the point where they're parallel to the floor.

GRIP
Take an overhand grip on the bar, your hands a comfortable distance apart.

MOVEMENT
Don't swing your legs behind you at the bottom to gather momentum for the next rep. Come to a full stop or have a partner slow your momentum after each rep.

SPEED
Use a controlled motion; swinging your body robs your abs of the workload.

POSITION
Bend your hips slightly at the bottom.

ANGLES
Bend your knees 90 degrees and lock them in this position for the entire set.

MOVEMENT
Think of curling your spine from the bottom up, not simply lifting your knees. You want the lower portion of your glutes to curl up at the top.

A

B

[FASTFACT]

This is a good exercise to perform first in your ab routine. Try it last and you'll notice how few reps you can complete with good form.

MAKE IT HARDER

Extend your legs to lengthen the lever and increase the resistance. Try doing as many reps as you can with straightened legs, then bend your knees to complete a few more reps.

[TIP08]

Use ab straps if your grip starts to give out before your abs do. That way you can take your sets to failure.

SKILL LEVEL

3

Vertical-Bench Knee Raise

This movement stabilizes your upper body better than the hanging version, so you can focus more intensely on your lower abs. You also won't worry about your grip giving out before your abs do.

POSITION
Allow your lower body to hang freely, back and glutes lightly touching the backpad.

GRIP
Grasp the handles with your forearms on the pads.

ANGLES
Bend your knees about 90 degrees and lock them in this position for the entire set.

POSITION
Bend your hips at the bottom.

MOVEMENT
Come to a full stop at the bottom of each rep. Don't swing your legs behind you to gather momentum for the next rep.

FORM
Lift your knees well above the point where they're parallel to the floor.

BREATH
Exhale as you reach the top position.

MOVEMENT
Use your abs to bring your knees as high as you can into your chest.

SPEED
Use a controlled motion; swinging your body robs your abs of the workload.

MOVEMENT
Think of curling your spine from the bottom up, not simply lifting your knees. You want the lower portion of your glutes to curl up from the pad.

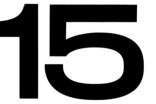
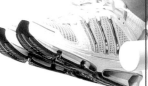

A

B

SKILL LEVEL
3

[**FASTFACT**]
Your lower abs really kick in when you bring your knees past the horizontal plane. If you consistently fail to go above this point, the exercise focuses more on your hip flexors.

15 If you can do more than **15 reps** with good form, fully straighten your legs to increase the degree of difficulty.

[**TIP09**]
Consciously try to get your glutes off the pad by bringing your knees as high as possible. This curls your hips up to rotate your pelvis, which is vital for lower-ab training.

Reverse Crunch on Incline Board

Get off the floor to make the standard reverse crunch a tougher move.

POSITION
Lie back on the bench with your head, shoulders and back firmly supported.

POSITION
Grasp the end of the bench with both hands.

ANGLES
Bend your hips and knees about 90 degrees and lift your feet off the floor.

SETUP
Place the incline board at the appropriate angle. Start at about 30 degrees and go steeper for more difficulty.

BREATH
Exhale after you reach the top position.

FORM
Keep your legs locked in the bent-knee position throughout the set.

A

B

SPEED
Use a controlled motion on both the positive and negative portions of the rep.

MOVEMENT
Curl your knees toward your chest by contracting your abs to lift your glutes fully off the pad.

SKILL LEVEL

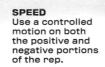

3

[FASTFACT]

Start your lower-ab workout with a tougher exercise like the reverse crunch on incline board. As you fatigue, choose less-challenging moves, such as those done on the floor.

MAKE IT HARDER

As you get stronger, set the incline bench to a steeper angle to continue making improvements in your muscle development. Decreasing the bend in your knees also increases the move's difficulty.

[TIP10]

Set the bench angle high and do as many reps as you can, then quickly get off and lower it one stop and continue the set, repeating this pattern until you reach the lowest position.

[LOWER]

Scissor Kick

This challenging move doesn't require any equipment, so you can do it at home.

POSITION
Extend your legs, keeping your heels about 6 inches off the floor to start. Maintain a very slight bend in your knees.

POSITION
To avoid hyperextending your neck, lift your head off the floor or place a pillow underneath it for support.

POSITION
Lie faceup with your arms by your sides, palms facing down.

A

BREATH
Hold your breath until you reach the top position to better stabilize your torso.

MOVEMENT
Make small, alternating, up-and-down scissorlike motions as you lift each leg.

FORM
Don't allow your heels to touch the floor at the bottom, which takes tension off your abs.

MOVEMENT
Raise your feet as you scissor them until they're about 45 degrees in the air.

SPEED
Use a rapid up-and-down motion in very short pulses as you raise your legs.

B

SKILL
LEVEL

3

[FASTFACT]

Keeping a slight bend in your knees, even on straight-legged movements, is a good idea because it reduces the force on your joints. Always do this when you extend your legs.

MAKE IT HARDER

Lie faceup on an incline board, grasping the end of the bench above your head. Perform the same movement, but bring your legs up to an even higher position relative to your body.

[TIP11]

While the pace of the scissor motion is fairly rapid, take two seconds total to complete the concentric (raising) action and another two for the eccentric (lowering) action.

Hip Thrust on Incline Board

The hip thrust may be hard, but adding the angled bench makes it more difficult. Try this when the floor version becomes too easy.

[FASTFACT]

Keep your legs perpendicular to the floor (not just to your body or the bench) to work your lower abs most efficiently.

12

When you can do **12 reps** with good form, increase the angle of the bench to further challenge your abs. Do three sets.

[TIP12]

This movement has a very small range of motion, which can best be measured by how far you get your glutes off the board. This is critical to recruiting your lower abs.

SETUP
Position the bench at the appropriate angle, about 30 degrees to start.

POSITION
Lie back on the bench with your head, shoulders and back firmly supported.

POSITION
Grasp the end of the bench or the handle at the top with both hands for support.

A

POSITION
Raise your legs so that your toes point at the ceiling. Your legs should be extended with just a slight bend in your knees.

MOVEMENT
Contract your abs to lift your glutes off the bench. They should rise at least 1–2 inches.

BREATH
Exhale after you reach the uppermost position.

B

MOVEMENT
Think about pressing your toes straight up into the ceiling.

SPEED
Control the motion; don't use body english to generate momentum. Your abs should drive the movement.

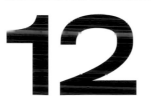

SKILL LEVEL

4

[LOWER]

Hanging Leg Raise

For advanced trainees, this is a good first movement to target the lower region of your abs. You likely won't be able to perform a high number of reps, so do it when you're fresh.

BREATH
Exhale as you reach the top position.

GRIP
Hold the bar with a wide overhand grip. If you use ab straps, keep them about shoulder-width apart.

A

FORM
Hold the peak-contracted position momentarily before going into the next rep.

MOVEMENT
Lower your legs under control, coming to a dead stop at the bottom of the rep. Don't swing your legs much past the plane of your body to gather momentum for the next rep. You should bring them back only slightly.

POSITION
Hang straight down, body fully extended, with a slight bend in your knees and hips and an arch in your lower back.

MOVEMENT
Keep your feet together as you use abdominal strength to raise your legs as high as possible — at least past parallel to the floor — without swinging your body.

FORM
You should have just a slight bend in your knees throughout.

POSITION
The lower portion of your glutes should curl up at the top to fully engage your lower abs, which occurs when you bring your legs above the parallel plane.

B

SKILL LEVEL

4

[FASTFACT]

Working in a lower rep range promotes ab strength and thickness. Choose moves with which you can complete more reps if you don't want to build up your midsection.

MAKE IT EASIER

If this version is too difficult or if you want to continue a set past muscle failure, increase the bend in your knees to decrease the resistance. Using ab straps can help you keep your grip on the bar.

[TIP 13]

It's easy to start swinging your body as you rack up the reps. If that happens, get a spotter to push against your lower back to prevent your body from moving back and forth.

[LOWER]

Vertical-Bench Leg Raise

It may be a bit easier than its hanging counterpart, but this advanced move will still make your midsection burn.

A

GRIP
Grasp the handles with your forearms on the pads.

FORM
Bend your hips very slightly at the bottom.

POSITION
Allow your lower body to hang freely, back and glutes lightly touching the backpad.

MOVEMENT
Come to a full stop at the bottom of the rep. Don't swing your legs behind you to gather momentum for the next rep.

MOVEMENT
Contract your abs to bring your feet as high as you possibly can.

MOVEMENT
Think of curling your spine from the bottom up, not simply lifting your legs. You want the lower portion of your glutes to curl up off the pad.

FORM
Fully extend your legs to just short of lockout to reduce pressure on your lower back and knee joints. Lock them in this position for the entire set.

FORM
Get your feet above the point where they're parallel to the floor to ensure contraction of your lower abs.

SPEED
Use a controlled motion; swinging your body robs your abs of the workload.

BREATH
Exhale as you reach the top position.

B

SKILL LEVEL

4

[FASTFACT]

[FASTFACT]

Lower-ab exercises require your pelvis to rotate, which occurs with motion in your lower glutes. They should come off the backpad as your hips curl at the top of the move.

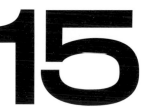

15

If you can do **15 reps**, try raising your feet higher, completely stopping between reps or reducing rest between sets.

[TIP14]

Once you hit muscle failure with the straight-leg version, bend your knees (and lock them in this position) to continue the set and rep to failure again.

[LOWER]

Lower-Ab Machine

SETUP
Adjust the machine to fit your torso length. Try repping with a very light weight to test the setting before beginning your sets.

POSITION
Grasp the handles overhead for support.

BREATH
Exhale only after reaching the peak-contracted position.

POSITION
Lie faceup in the machine with your head, back and shoulders square against the pads. If your unit has thigh straps, secure them around your thighs.

MOVEMENT
Don't allow the weights to touch the stack at the bottom of the rep, which takes the stress off the working muscles.

FORM
Your body should remain still during the movement; don't squirm in an effort to help assist in the lift.

This is essentially a reverse crunch done with added variable resistance. Use heavy weight and low reps for strength, or employ lighter weights and higher reps to work on endurance.

MOVEMENT
Contract your lower abs to bring your knees toward your chest as high as possible.

SPEED
Use a strong but smooth motion on the positive portion of the rep; lower the weights smoothly and under control.

SKILL LEVEL

4

[FASTFACT]
All moves in which you bring your knees toward your chest should be done through as full a range of motion as possible to optimally stress your lower-ab region. Don't do half-reps.

10

Once you can do **10 good reps,** add another plate and try for eight. Add more resistance when you reach 10 reps again.

[TIP15]
Try repping to failure with a very heavy weight. Immediately reduce the weight by two pins and go to failure again. Repeat in this manner until you reach failure with a very light weight.

Rocky IV

This one is sure to drop jaws at the gym. Make sure you do it correctly for safety, and get ready to field lots of questions about its origins.

POSITION
Lie faceup on a flat bench, your body extended and legs straight, knees bent slightly.

POSITION
Contract your abs to lift your entire torso off the bench to start. Only your shoulders and head should touch the bench throughout the movement.

POSITION
Grasp the edges of the bench overhead to firmly support your body.

A

BREATH
Exhale as you reach the top position.

MOVEMENT
Contract your abs to raise your entire body — legs, hips, lower and middle back — directly upward, straight toward the ceiling.

B

[FASTFACT]

This exercise was made popular — but not easy — in Sylvester Stallone's hit *Rocky* movies. No doubt the actor was in supreme shape when he made these flicks.

MAKE IT HARDER

Yes, it's possible. Do the same movement on an incline board (or decline bench, with your head at the top) to up the level of difficulty.

[TIP16]

You need exceptional ab strength to hold your body in this position, let alone control raising and lowering it. Try doing one rep right and build from there. Have a spotter on hand to help you with form.

SPEED
Use a smooth, controlled speed on both the ascent and descent. If you come down too fast, your glutes will hit the bench, taking the muscular stress off your abs.

FORM
Keep your body as straight as possible.

SKILL LEVEL

5

[UPPER]

Supported Crunch

You get better leverage with your feet pressed against a fixed object, enabling you to go a little higher and work your abs more efficiently.

A

POSITION
Your lower legs or heels should rest on the bench.

ANGLES
Your hip and knee joints should be bent about 90 degrees.

POSITION
Lightly cup your head with your hands.

POSITION
Your back and glutes should be on the floor.

B

SPEED
Move at a deliberate speed using only your ab strength, not momentum.

BREATH
Exhale as you reach the top position.

FORM
Keep your head neutrally aligned — neither pulled forward nor extended backward.

CAUTION
Don't pull on your head in an effort to get yourself up.

MOVEMENT
Curl your shoulder blades off the floor, going as high as you can.

SKILL LEVEL

2

[FASTFACT]
Crunches use a relatively small range of motion — your shoulder blades move only a few inches. Squeeze your abs at the peak-contracted position at the top of the rep.

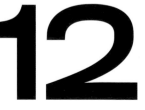

If you can do more than **12 reps** with good form, challenge your abs by adding weight or taking a shorter rest period.

[TIP17]
It's all about getting your shoulder blades off the mat. For a more intense workout, don't touch bottom at the end of the rep to maintain tension on your abs.

Exercise-Ball Crunch

Get off the floor and do your crunches on an exercise ball for an increased range of motion and better development.

POSITION
Your hands should lightly support your head.

MOVEMENT
Crunch your upper body forward, rolling your shoulders toward your hips. Bring your shoulder blades off the ball as high as possible.

MOVEMENT
On the descent, go past the point where you'd normally stop when crunching on the floor. This fully stretches your abs and increases the range of motion.

A

POSITION
Sit on top of a fairly large exercise ball and slide forward, rolling the bottom half of your glutes off the ball.

POSITION
Place your feet shoulder–width apart or wider on the floor.

MOVEMENT
Squeeze your abs at the point of peak contraction for a full second before lowering.

B

FORM
Think of pressing your lower back hard into the ball to help bring your shoulder blades up.

SPEED
Perform your reps slowly and smoothly. You're not racing to complete a number of reps but rather trying to feel your abs working on each and every rep.

[FASTFACT]

Because of their relative instability, exercise balls call additional stabilizer muscles into play, making this move more difficult than its floor– or bench–crunch counterparts.

MAKE IT HARDER
Carefully hold a dumbbell or small weight plate behind your head to increase the resistance. Take advantage of the prestretch the ball allows by extending back over it as far as you can.

[TIP18]

By rotating one elbow toward the opposite knee at the top of the movement, you can recruit your obliques. Alternate sides or do all your reps for one side first before switching.

[UPPER]

SKILL
LEVEL

2

Crunch (Hands Overhead)

Extend your arms to add an element of instability and increase the resistance of this short crunching motion.

FORM
Keep your head neutrally aligned; look up at the ceiling to avoid pressing your chin into your chest.

BREATH
Exhale as you reach the top position.

MOVEMENT
Contract your abs to lift your shoulder blades off the floor.

POSITION
Lie flat on the floor with a 60-degree bend in your knees.

POSITION
Extend your arms overhead, crossing your palms.

POSITION
Your feet should be flat on the floor, shoulder-width apart.

FORM
Consciously press your lower back into the floor to help get your shoulder blades higher off the mat.

FORM
Keep your arms aligned with your head, neck, shoulders and spine.

MOVEMENT
Don't let your head touch the floor, and try to stop short of fully supporting your upper body on the mat to maintain tension on your abs.

[UPPER]

SKILL LEVEL

2

[FASTFACT]

Moving your arms away from the axis of rotation near your hips ups the resistance. Test the degree of difficulty by placing your hands on your hips, across your chest and overhead.

15

If you can do more than **15 reps** using a controlled pace, it's time you switched to a more challenging upper-ab movement.

[TIP19]

As you fatigue during the arms-overhead version, quickly reposition your arms across your chest or alongside your hips to take the set to total failure.

Tuck Crunch

This challenging move recruits the lower abs but focuses on the upper portion of the rectus abdominis.

POSITION
Lie on the floor with your hands crossed over your chest.

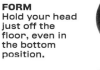

A

ANGLES
Bend your knees and hips to form right angles, keeping your lower legs parallel to the floor and your ankles crossed.

FORM
Hold your head just off the floor, even in the bottom position.

BREATH
Exhale at the top of the movement.

FORM
Your legs remain stationary throughout the rep.

B

MOVEMENT
Curl up to lift your shoulder blades a few inches off the floor.

FORM
Hold the peak-contracted position for a long second to increase the intensity and feel your abs contract.

SPEED
Use a smooth motion as you crunch up; don't jerk your head up in an effort to build momentum to help you rise.

[UPPER]

[FASTFACT]

Supporting your legs in the air requires your lower abs to work isometrically, while your upper abs work dynamically by contracting through a range of motion.

MAKE IT HARDER

Cup your hands behind your head to support it (but avoid pulling on it), or you can really boost the resistance by carefully holding a small weight plate or dumbbell behind your head.

[TIP20]

Crunch your upper body forward while simultaneously doing a reverse crunch with your lower body. This double crunch works both ends of the rectus abdominis.

SKILL LEVEL

Straight-Leg Crunch

Though this isn't considered a lower-ab movement, your lower abs isometrically contract to hold your legs in position.

[UPPER]

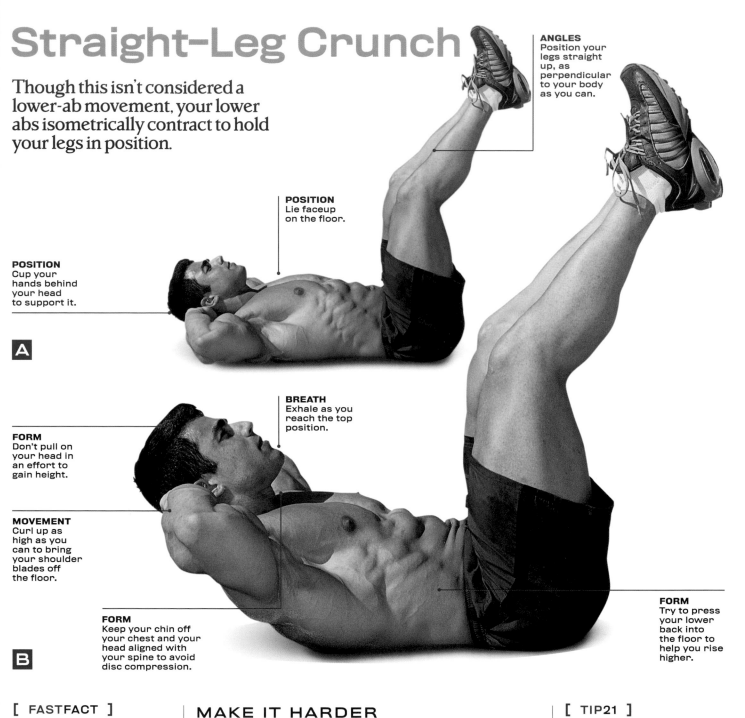

ANGLES
Position your legs straight up, as perpendicular to your body as you can.

POSITION
Lie faceup on the floor.

POSITION
Cup your hands behind your head to support it.

A

BREATH
Exhale as you reach the top position.

FORM
Don't pull on your head in an effort to gain height.

MOVEMENT
Curl up as high as you can to bring your shoulder blades off the floor.

FORM
Keep your chin off your chest and your head aligned with your spine to avoid disc compression.

FORM
Try to press your lower back into the floor to help you rise higher.

B

SKILL LEVEL

2

[FASTFACT]

To make any ab exercise harder, hold the top position for a second. This requires you to hold the peak contraction, rather than just releasing and returning to the start.

MAKE IT HARDER

The whole idea is to get your shoulder blades a little farther off the mat. Try to go higher on each rep while still controlling the motion and avoiding the use of muscle-robbing momentum.

[TIP21]

Keeping your legs upright is fairly difficult, so make sure you train your lower abs regularly by starting with easier leg positions, like the tuck, before progressing to this one.

Crunch on Back-Extension Bench

 A

FORM
Lie back, using your abs to control the descent, till your body is in one linear plane.

POSITION
Place your feet under the rollers, slightly flexing your ankles to maintain your body position.

POSITION
Your glutes should sit back toward the top of the bench, legs straight.

POSITION
Lightly support your head with your hands.

BREATH
Exhale as you reach the point of peak contraction.

ANGLES
You don't need to go much past 45 degrees to get full abdominal contraction. In fact, going too high might allow your abs to rest as your body approaches perpendicular.

MOVEMENT
Contract your abs to curl your torso up.

B

FORM
For better contraction, round your back as you squeeze your abs.

SPEED
Control both the positive and negative motion. This is especially critical on the return to prevent hyperextending your back.

[**FASTFACT**]

You can use the back-extension bench to perform a challenging tri-set consisting of the crunches pictured here, oblique crunches and back extensions.

MAKE IT HARDER

Hold a weight plate across your chest or behind your head. After you fatigue, drop it and keep going to failure.

[**TIP22**]

When your feet are anchored, as in this exercise, your hip-flexor muscles assist in the movement. In such cases, round your back as you curl up to increase the contribution from your abdominals.

This bench can work both your abs and low back with a simple change of body position. Training your lower back ensures that your core has no weak areas, which helps prevent injury in the long run.

[UPPER]

SKILL LEVEL

2

Decline-Bench Crunch

Opt for this underutilized bench when the gym's ab equipment is being used. By adjusting the angle, it can be good for beginners to advanced trainees.

[UPPER]

MOVEMENT
Stop about two-thirds of the way down to stretch your abs before going into the next rep.

POSITION
Place your hands behind your head or cross them over your chest, which makes the exercise slightly easier.

A

POSITION
Secure your feet under the ankle pads.

FORM
Round your back to increase the abdominal contraction as you rise.

MOVEMENT
Contract your abs to curl your body up to a point about perpendicular to the bench. You don't need to go all the way to perpendicular to the floor.

SPEED
Use a smooth, controlled motion on both the up and down phases.

FORM
Your hip flexors are highly activated during this movement, so try not to squeeze your quads to pull through your legs.

B

SKILL LEVEL

3

[FASTFACT]

You can turn many upper-ab moves into combination exercises that also train the obliques. Just aim one shoulder toward the opposite knee as you come up, then switch.

MAKE IT HARDER

Increase the angle of the bench. If using a steep decline isn't enough, carefully hold a small weight plate against your chest or behind your head to really challenge your abs.

[TIP23]

Start with a steep decline and, as your abs become fatigued, decrease the angle as you do more sets. This gives you a thorough upper-ab workout on one piece of equipment.

Weighted medicine balls help you progressively overload your upper abs, and your partner can push you to perform more sets.

Medicine-Ball Crunch

SETUP
Your partner should stand 5–8 feet away in the "ready" position (when not throwing).

MOVEMENT
Catch the ball in the up position and return to the floor.

FORM
Use a two-handed chest pass to toss the ball to your partner once you're almost at the top position.

MOVEMENT
Use your abs to rise as high as you can. Your shoulder blades should come way off the floor.

BREATH
Exhale as you reach the top position and pass the ball.

[UPPER]

A

B

POSITION
Lie faceup with your knees bent and feet flat on the floor. Your hands should be in front of you in the "ready" position as you prepare to toss/catch the ball.

SPEED
Don't "bounce" off the floor to generate momentum for the next rep. Reverse direction deliberately and smoothly using only your abs.

SKILL LEVEL

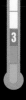

3

[FASTFACT]

Medicine-ball workouts are decidedly old school, but an entire routine of such crunches can really shake up your routine. Put several together and see how sore you get.

MAKE IT HARDER

Switch to a heavier medicine ball or perform this exercise on a decline bench to increase the level of difficulty. Try not to pull through your legs when on the bench — try to maintain tension on your abs.

[TIP24]

Do this move last in your workout. Training with a partner could help you get more reps than you would on your own. See if you can really work through the burn.

Exercise-Ball Crunch With Rope

GRIP
Grasp the rope, holding the ends alongside your head. Keep this position throughout.

POSITION
Place your feet flat on the floor to maintain balance.

FORM
Keep your hands near your ears as you crunch so your arms can't assist in raising the weight stack.

A

SETUP
Position an exercise ball about 2 feet away from a low-cable pulley.

POSITION
Sit atop the exercise ball and roll the bottom half of your glutes off the ball till your back is firmly on top of the ball.

This move has it all: a great prestretch, a balance component to challenge your core muscles and the benefit of added resistance to hit your abs hard.

MOVEMENT
Get your shoulder blades as high off the ball as possible. Hold the peak-contracted position for a second before reversing direction.

MOVEMENT
Squeeze your abs and curl forward.

FORM
Press your lower back into the ball to help you rise as high as you can.

B

SKILL LEVEL

4

[FASTFACT]

This is a smart way to overload your abs when bodyweight-only exercises aren't enough. Try 6-8 reps for strength, 10-12 for muscle-building and 15-plus for muscular endurance.

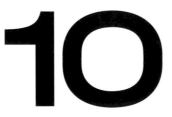

10

Once you can do **10 reps** with good form, add a plate to the stack. This is more challenging than simply adding reps.

[TIP25]

Minimizing arm movement is critical to keeping the focus on your abs. Lock your hands by the sides of your head to force your abs to pull up the weight.

Lying Cable Crunch

This exercise is a cross between the tried-and-true floor crunch and the cable crunch. It allows advanced-level trainees to significantly increase the resistance.

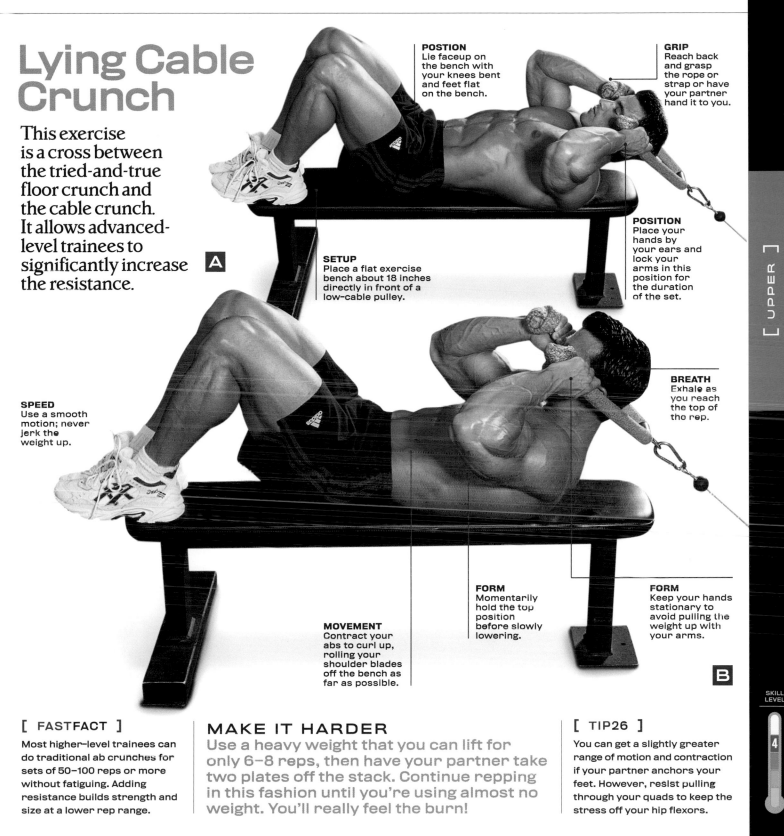

POSTION
Lie faceup on the bench with your knees bent and feet flat on the bench.

GRIP
Reach back and grasp the rope or strap or have your partner hand it to you.

SETUP
Place a flat exercise bench about 18 inches directly in front of a low-cable pulley.

A

POSITION
Place your hands by your ears and lock your arms in this position for the duration of the set.

SPEED
Use a smooth motion; never jerk the weight up.

BREATH
Exhale as you reach the top of the rep.

MOVEMENT
Contract your abs to curl up, rolling your shoulder blades off the bench as far as possible.

FORM
Momentarily hold the top position before slowly lowering.

FORM
Keep your hands stationary to avoid pulling the weight up with your arms.

B

[UPPER]

SKILL LEVEL

4

[FASTFACT]

Most higher-level trainees can do traditional ab crunches for sets of 50–100 reps or more without fatiguing. Adding resistance builds strength and size at a lower rep range.

MAKE IT HARDER

Use a heavy weight that you can lift for only 6–8 reps, then have your partner take two plates off the stack. Continue repping in this fashion until you're using almost no weight. You'll really feel the burn!

[TIP26]

You can get a slightly greater range of motion and contraction if your partner anchors your feet. However, resist pulling through your quads to keep the stress off your hip flexors.

Cable Crunch

As you get stronger, you can selectively increase the resistance to continue making gains in your desired rep range.

[UPPER]

SETUP
Attach a rope or strap to a high-cable pulley and select the appropriate resistance.

GRIP
Firmly grasp the rope attachment with both hands.

POSITION
Place your hands by your ears and lock your hands and arms in this position for the duration of the set.

MOVEMENT
You don't need to come up to a completely vertical position to stretch your abs.

MOVEMENT
Contract your abs to bring your elbows toward the floor in an arc as far as you can.

FORM
Your back must round for this move to effectively target your abdominals.

FORM
Keep your head neutrally aligned. Don't tuck your chin into your chest at any time.

A

POSITION
Kneel about 2–3 feet from and facing a high-cable pulley.

FORM
Don't let your glutes shift back. Think of your hips as a hinge with the only movement taking place in your upper torso.

B

BREATH
Exhale when you're at the lowest point.

SKILL LEVEL

4

[FASTFACT]

Because you can go very heavy with these, cable crunches are a smart choice for the first exercise in an advanced trainee's upper-ab routine.

MAKE IT HARDER

Have your partner watch your form; most people accidentally sit back as they crunch forward, which makes the move easier. Keep the action confined to the abdominals by locking all other joints in place.

[TIP27]

Rounding your back is critical when training abs, but avoid pressing your chin into your chest. Imagine a tennis ball is lodged between the two to keep your head in proper position.

Machine Crunch

The keys to this exercise are to feel your abs draw your pelvis and ribcage together and squeeze momentarily at the point of peak contraction.

SETUP
Adjust the seat back and resistance according to your needs. Sit snugly in the machine.

MOVEMENT
As you return to the start position, don't allow the weight stack to hit bottom, which releases tension on your abs.

FORM
Keep your head neutrally aligned; don't press your chin into your chest in an effort to help you press the resistance pad downward.

FORM
Your back should round as you complete the movement. Visualize your abdominal wall contracting section by section.

MOVEMENT
Contract your abs to press your chest against the pad so your spine flexes forward.

FORM
Avoid pulling through your quads and hip flexors to assist in the movement.

SPEED
Use a smooth motion at all times. Control both the positive and negative portions of each rep.

POSITION
Place your feet under the rollers.

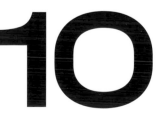

A

B

[UPPER]

SKILL LEVEL

4

[FASTFACT]

Ab machines vary by manufacturer, and some may feel smoother than others. Try various machines and see which ones fit your body best and feel right to you.

10

If your goal is to build muscle and you can do more than **10 reps** with good form, simply increase the weight next time.

[TIP28]

Because the weight is easily adjusted, machines can be useful for beginning to advanced trainees. Set the resistance to match your goals: strength, size or endurance.

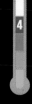

Medicine-Ball Twist

Bring a friend to the gym to make your ab training more productive and fun.

MOVEMENT
As you receive the ball from your partner, twist fully in the opposite direction, feeling the movement in your obliques.

A

POSITION
Stand erect and plant your feet shoulder-width apart.

SETUP
Stand 6–8 feet away from your partner, sides facing each other.

B

GRIP
Hold the weighted medicine ball with both hands in front of you.

BREATH
Exhale as you pass the ball.

SPEED
Use your obliques, not your arms, to generate the force to twist and toss the ball. Your obliques should power the twist, not momentum.

MOVEMENT
Twist toward your partner and toss him/her the ball as he/she begins to twist toward you.

OBLIQUES

SKILL LEVEL

2

[FASTFACT]
Oblique training involves trunk rotation (twisting from side to side) as opposed to spinal flexion (bringing the pelvis and ribcage closer together, as in crunching movements).

MAKE IT HARDER
Try using a slightly heavier medicine ball. Beware of increasing the speed of the movement by using momentum; use a smooth, controlled tempo to really feel your obliques working and to avoid injury.

[TIP29]
When you catch the ball, you can exaggerate the twist for greater effect on your muscles. Remember to switch places with your partner to work both sides of your body.

Side Bend

Working your obliques in the lateral plane is easy to do. It's also easy to increase resistance — just add more weight.

B

POSITION
Your back should be flat and your head focused forward.

POSITION
Stand erect with your feet shoulder-width apart and your knees straight but not locked.

BREATH
Exhale as you reach the down position.

MOVEMENT
Using the power generated by your obliques, crunch down in the opposite direction.

MOVEMENT
Bend laterally toward the weighted hand.

FORM
Keep the movement confined to the lateral plane, not forward or backward.

SPEED
Use a controlled yet powerful motion.

GRIP
One hand should hold a weighted dumbbell; place the other behind your head.

[OBLIQUES]

SKILL LEVEL

2

[FASTFACT]

Many people who don't want to build thicker, muscular obliques avoid using heavy weights and instead perform this exercise with little or no weight for high reps.

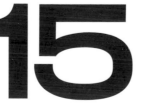

If you want to add size and you can do more than about **15 reps** with good form, add weight to the dumbbell.

[TIP30]

This move's range of motion is fairly small. Feel the contraction of your obliques in the bottom position and hold it momentarily. Don't forget to work both sides of your body.

Standing Rotation

Here's another way to incorporate a standing oblique exercise into your routine to complement those you do lying down and more thoroughly work your abs.

B

A

GRIP
Hold the medicine ball with both hands in front of your forehead.

MOVEMENT
Rotate your torso to one side and pass the ball high to your partner, who has simultaneously rotated toward you.

MOVEMENT
Rotate in the opposite direction and receive the ball back from your partner.

POSITION
Stand about 6 inches from your workout partner, back to back. Plant your feet and keep them there.

FORM
This time, you receive the ball in a lower position (hands at your waist rather than at shoulder level).

POSITION
Stand up straight to start, knees slightly bent.

SPEED
This is not a race. You should feel the power of your obliques working to rotate your torso.

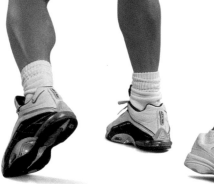

OBLIQUES

SKILL LEVEL

2

[FASTFACT]
Do ab exercises with a partner once a week to introduce new moves that target your muscles a little differently — a smart way to more thoroughly work your midsection.

MAKE IT HARDER
Try it with a heavier medicine ball, but be especially aware of keeping the movement smooth and controlled. You want to most efficiently work your obliques and at the same time prevent injury.

[TIP31]
Keep your lower body as still as possible so your obliques do the work to rotate your body from side to side. Don't forget to train the opposite side of your body in the same manner.

Oblique Crunch on Angled Back-Extension Bench

Envision the side bend done at an angle, and you've got this bench-supported version that really whittles your middle.

BREATH
Exhale as you reach the top position.

POSITION
Cup your head with one hand; the other should touch your abs.

FORM
In the bottom position, your upper body should be bent sideways at the waist (not angled forward or backward).

POSITION
Place your outer thigh against the pad so that you face sideways.

MOVEMENT
Contract your obliques to curl your body in the opposite direction, rising as high as you can.

FORM
Stay in the lateral plane.

SPEED
Use a deliberate, smooth motion.

SETUP
Adjust the height of the bench so your torso can bend freely from your hips.

POSITION
Place both ankles under the rollers on the bench.

A

B

[OBLIQUES]

SKILL LEVEL

2

[FASTFACT]

Because you're working more against gravity, using an angled bench forces your obliques to work a little harder than they do on the upright side bend. Work both sides.

MAKE IT HARDER

Grasp a lightweight dumbbell in your free hand and allow your arm to hang straight toward the floor. Make sure you control the negative rep rather than just letting the weight pull you down.

[TIP32]

You can also perform this exercise faceup by adding a twisting motion to each side, which recruits your upper abs in addition to your obliques.

Oblique Crunch on Back-Extension Bench

The back-extension bench anchors your feet, enabling you to go higher than moves in which your feet aren't secured. This results in a stronger contraction.

POSITION
Cup your head with your top hand to support it.

SETUP
Adjust the bench so that the front and rear pads are approximately the same height.

POSITION
Place your outer thigh against the bench so that you face sideways.

MOVEMENT
Curl your torso up as high as possible in the lateral plane, contracting your obliques hard at the top.

POSITION
Place both feet under the rear pad.

FORM
Don't go past parallel to the floor when you descend.

POSITION
Your hips should be free to move, hanging just off the end of the bench.

SPEED
Use a smooth and deliberate motion on the up phase, and control the negative.

OBLIQUES

SKILL LEVEL

3

[FASTFACT]
When training obliques, squeeze the muscles hard at the top of the movement, feeling the contraction and holding it momentarily before releasing and returning to the start.

MAKE IT HARDER
Carefully hold a small weight plate or dumbbell behind your head to increase the resistance.

[TIP33]
You can also perform this exercise faceup by adding a twisting motion to each side, which works your upper abs as well as your obliques. Remember to train both sides.

Rotary Machine Twist

You can progressively increase the weight over time to overload your obliques for continued gains in muscle and strength.

SETUP
Adjust the machine for resistance and body measurements.

POSITION
Place your arms firmly against the pads. Lock your arms in position for the duration of the set.

POSITION
Sit upright against the backpad. Keep your head aligned with your body as your upper torso rotates.

MOVEMENT
Use your obliques to twist at the hips as far as you can go, holding the peak contraction for a count before releasing. Twist back in the opposite direction to work both sides.

FORM
Don't use your arm strength to assist in the movement. Contract only through your obliques.

SPEED
Use a forceful contraction that's smooth and controlled; don't use momentum or push through your arms to rotate from side to side.

POSITION
Touch your feet to the floor to better stabilize your body.

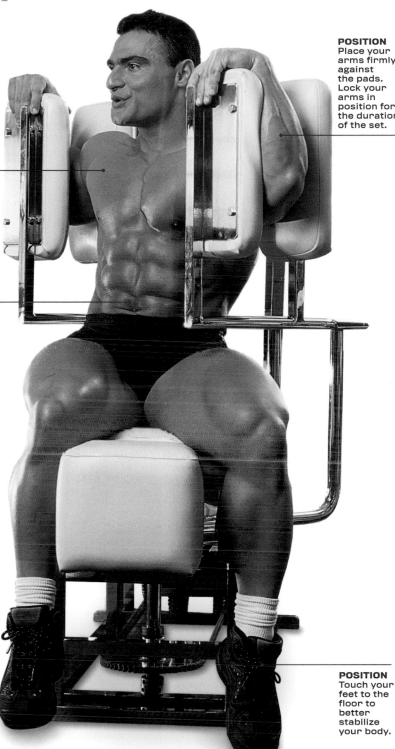

[**FASTFACT**]

Most oblique exercises involve crunching to the sides in a lateral plane, but twisting moves rotate your torso at the waist. Use both types in your oblique training.

MAKE IT HARDER

Try this drop set: Go very heavy for as many reps as you can do (choose a weight with which you can do no more than about 12), then quickly drop the weight by two plates and resume your set, continuing in this fashion for several drop sets.

[**TIP34**]

Twisting movements are easy to cheat on by using momentum instead of muscle. That's why holding the twist position and forcefully contracting your muscle at this point helps you to more efficiently work your obliques.

OBLIQUES

SKILL LEVEL

3

Side Leg Raise

This is an advanced version of the oblique crunch in which both ends of your body rise simultaneously for a stronger contraction along the entire muscle.

OBLIQUES

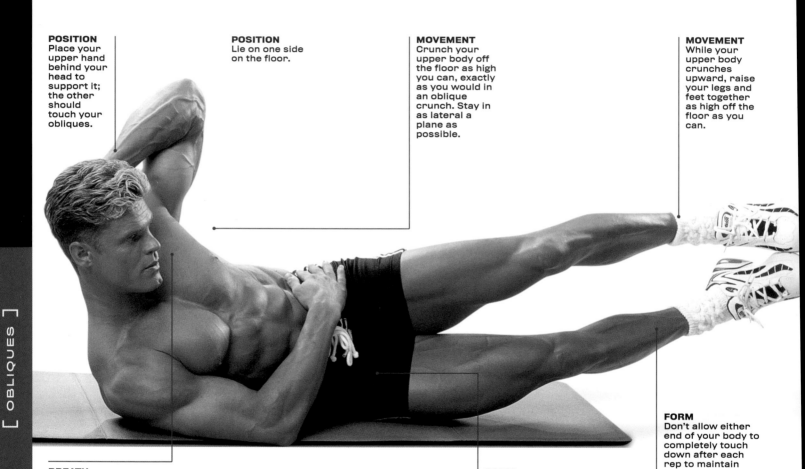

POSITION
Place your upper hand behind your head to support it; the other should touch your obliques.

POSITION
Lie on one side on the floor.

MOVEMENT
Crunch your upper body off the floor as high you can, exactly as you would in an oblique crunch. Stay in as lateral a plane as possible.

MOVEMENT
While your upper body crunches upward, raise your legs and feet together as high off the floor as you can.

BREATH
Exhale as both ends of your body reach the top position.

FORM
Your knees and hips should be just slightly bent.

FORM
Don't allow either end of your body to completely touch down after each rep to maintain constant tension on your muscles throughout the set.

SKILL LEVEL

3

[FASTFACT]

In most oblique exercises, you crunch your upper body in the lateral plane down toward your same-side leg, but this is one of the few exercises in which your legs also move.

MAKE IT HARDER

You can choose from three intensity-boosting options: Hold the top position for a two-count, move slowly to fight the negative portion of the rep, or squeeze your obliques extra-hard.

[TIP35]

Rising as high as you can with both your upper body and legs is the key to really feeling your obliques contract along their whole length. Make sure you work both sides of your body.

Exercise-Ball Twist

Work your core muscles and stabilizers with this hard-hitting exercise-ball movement.

POSITION
Sit on an exercise ball with your feet flat on the floor. Place a dumbbell on your chest and roll your body forward until only your head and shoulders touch the ball.

GRIP
Raise the dumbbell over your chest until you lock out your arms.

FORM
Keep your head in normal alignment — don't flex it forward or extend it backward.

MOVEMENT
Twist your body to one side, beginning the rotation from your hips. Your lower body should not move.

POSITION
Straighten and tighten your lower back and raise your hips so they're only slightly lower than your shoulders.

MOVEMENT
Twist your torso until your arms are again parallel to the floor. Hold the position momentarily, then twist to the opposite side.

A

FORM
Allow your head to follow your hands.

SPEED
Use a smooth, controlled motion; you'll lose your balance on the ball if momentum takes over.

B

[OBLIQUES]

SKILL LEVEL

3

[FASTFACT]
Exercises that use added resistance, like a dumbbell in this case, can be tailored for everyone from beginners to advanced trainees simply by adjusting the weight.

MAKE IT HARDER
Link 3–4 exercise-ball movements, one each for upper and lower abs and obliques, in succession with no rest in between, for a killer tri-set. Rest only after you perform all the exercises, then repeat.

[TIP36]
Don't use any weight the first couple of times you try this exercise to learn the proper form. Once you get the hang of the movement, begin adding weight for continued gains.

Cable Woodchop

Experienced woodchoppers know that true power emanates from the core, and that's exactly how you do this exercise to achieve maximum results.

B

A

POSITION
Stand alongside the high-cable pulley with your right shoulder closest to the apparatus.

MOVEMENT
Using your left obliques to power the move, pull the handle down in an arc using your left arm to a position even with your left hip as your torso rotates at the waist.

BREATH
Exhale as you reach the bottom position.

FORM
Keep your lead (left) arm as straight as possible to keep the focus on your obliques. Your head should follow your hands.

GRIP
Reach your left arm across your body and grasp the handle. Place your right hand on top of your left. Keep both arms straight but unlocked throughout the set.

POSITION
Place your feet about shoulder-width apart and bend your knees slightly.

MOVEMENT
Hold the contraction briefly at the bottom, then return along the same arc to the start position.

OBLIQUES

SKILL LEVEL
3

[FASTFACT]
Choose a heavy weight with which you can do 4–6 reps for strength, slightly lighter weight for 8–12 reps to develop size, and very light weight for 15-plus reps to boost endurance.

MAKE IT HARDER
Add more weight to the stack as your skill with this movement improves and you can do 12–15 reps with good form. Try holding the peak-contracted position for a two-count while squeezing your obliques.

[TIP37]
Don't let your arms bend and extend to assist in the movement. Lock them into place and make your obliques work to pull the handle across your body. Work both sides.

Standing Oblique Cable Crunch

This is a good isolation movement that you can perform for high reps to carve detail into your obliques.

A

GRIP
Use an underhand grip with D-handle. Bend your arm to about 90 degrees, with your upper arm parallel to the floor. Lock it in this position for the duration of the set.

POSITION
Stand at about a 45-degree angle 2 feet away from a high-cable pulley, your right shoulder closest to the pulley.

BREATH
Exhale at the bottom.

POSITION
Place your feet shoulder-width apart and bend your knees slightly.

FORM
Your head should follow your hands and torso.

FORM
Keep your arm locked in position so it doesn't assist in the movement.

SPEED
Use a forceful but smooth speed on the positive motion and control the negative to more thoroughly work your muscle.

MOVEMENT
Using just your obliques, crunch down in the lateral plane as far as you can go. Hold the contraction for a count before releasing.

B

SKILL LEVEL

4

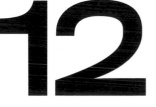

[**FASTFACT**]

You can perform most cable exercises for obliques in either a standing or kneeling position. Try both ways to find out which is more comfortable — and effective — for you.

12

If you can do more than **12 reps** on each side with good form, add weight to continue making gains in muscle size and strength.

[**TIP38**]

Try touching your obliques with your free hand to better feel them moving and to make sure you're not cheating on the rep. Remember to train both sides.

SKILL
LEVEL

2

Double Crunch

Work both the upper and lower ends of your
rectus abdominis with this two-sided move.

POSITION
Start in the
tuck-crunch
position with
your back flat
on the floor,
knees and
feet up.

ANGLES
Bend your knees and hips
to about 90-degree angles.
Lock your knees in this
position for the duration
of the set.

A

POSITION
Your hands
should lightly
support
your head,
just off the
floor to
start.

BREATH
Exhale as you
reach the top
position.

MOVEMENT
At the same
time, contract
your abs to
bring your
knees over your
chest and the
lower portion of
your glutes off
the floor.

MOVEMENT
Curl up as high as you
can, trying to bring
your shoulder blades
off the floor.

SPEED
Use a smooth
motion as your
ribcage and
hips move
toward each
other
simultaneously.

B

COMBOS

[FASTFACT]
You stimulate your upper abs
when you lift your shoulder
blades off the floor; you target
your lower abs when you bring
your knees over your chest
and curl your glutes up a bit.

MAKE IT HARDER
Rise as high as you can on both ends and
hold the peak contraction for a long count
before releasing. Feel your abs contract
and stretch on each rep rather than
counting numbers.

[TIP39]
Don't touch down at any point
during the set — you'll only
maintain continuous tension on
your abs by keeping both your
feet and head off the floor
between reps.

SKILL LEVEL

2

Scissor to a Crunch

This slightly more difficult version of the double crunch has an extra move to work your lower abs.

POSITION
Place your hands lightly behind your head to support it.

POSITION
Lie faceup on the floor with your legs out straight.

POSITION
Hold your heels about 6 inches off the floor to start.

A

MOVEMENT
Separate your legs as far apart as possible, then move them back together, but don't cross them.

B

FORM
The only movement thus far takes place in your lower body.

BREATH
Exhale at the top of the movement.

MOVEMENT
At the same time, curl up as high as you can, trying to get your shoulder blades off the floor.

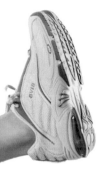

MOVEMENT
Once your legs are back together, bring your knees over your chest and the lower portion of your glutes off the floor.

C

[FASTFACT]

To keep tension on your abs, never allow your head or feet to come into contact with the floor during a set. That would allow the muscles involved to rest between reps.

MAKE IT HARDER

Do this as the last exercise in your ab workout, when your midsection is already fairly fatigued, to really incite a burn in your muscles.

[TIP40]

To better recruit your lower-abdominal region, focus on getting the lower portion of your glutes to come off the floor as you bring your knees over your chest.

[COMBOS]

SKILL LEVEL
2

Crossover Split-Leg Crunch

POSITION
Space your legs about 2 feet apart.

A

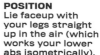

POSITION
Lie faceup with your legs straight up in the air (which works your lower abs isometrically).

POSITION
Place your hands lightly behind your head to support it, just off the floor to start.

B

FORM
Don't just flap your elbow across and think you're working your obliques. Make sure you rotate and turn one shoulder toward the opposite foot.

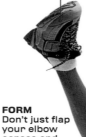

MOVEMENT
Curl your torso up, rotating one elbow and shoulder toward your opposite foot. Lower and repeat to the other side.

BREATH
Exhale at the top of the movement.

This is an advanced version of the crossover crunch in which you extend your legs into the air, which really challenges your lower abs.

SPEED
Use a smooth, controlled motion — don't jerk on your head in an effort to go higher.

[FASTFACT]

When you hold your lower abs in one position throughout a rep, you're training them isometrically. Your upper abs, on the other hand, contract over a larger range of motion.

MAKE IT HARDER
Instead of alternating sides, perform a rep to your left side, then do one straight up to your middle, then rep to your right side. Repeat this pattern back and forth to really challenge your midsection.

[TIP41]

You can also perform this exercise by extending your hands toward the toes of one foot, lowering and then repeating this motion toward your other foot.

COMBOS

SKILL
LEVEL

2

Figure 4 Crunch

Here's another tough bodyweight move that incorporates both the upper- and lower-ab regions.

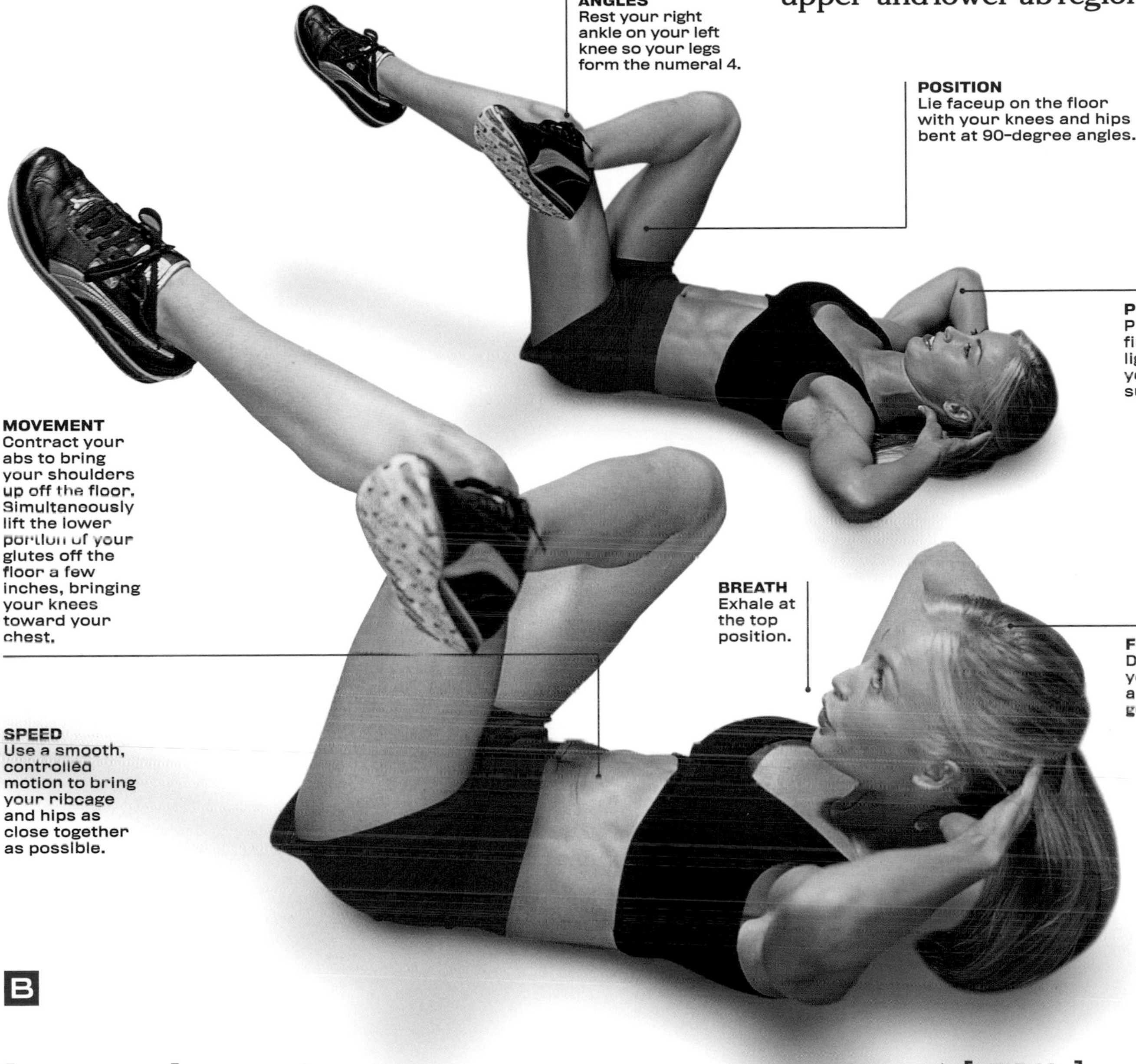

ANGLES
Rest your right ankle on your left knee so your legs form the numeral 4.

POSITION
Lie faceup on the floor with your knees and hips bent at 90–degree angles.

A

POSITION
Place your fingertips lightly behind your head to support it.

MOVEMENT
Contract your abs to bring your shoulders up off the floor. Simultaneously lift the lower portion of your glutes off the floor a few inches, bringing your knees toward your chest.

BREATH
Exhale at the top position.

FORM
Don't pull on your head in an effort to go higher.

SPEED
Use a smooth, controlled motion to bring your ribcage and hips as close together as possible.

B

[FASTFACT]

To work your lower abs most effectively, you need the lower portion of your glutes to curl up off the floor in the top position of this exercise.

MAKE IT HARDER

Bring in your obliques by rotating one shoulder and elbow toward the opposite foot. Add even more variety by alternating reps that go to the left side, straight up the middle and to the right side.

[TIP42]

Try to fold your body in half by pressing your spine into the floor and consciously closing the distance between your ribcage and your hips. Work both sides.

COMBOS

Alternate Twisting Exercise-Ball Crunch

Add a twist to the exercise-ball crunch to recruit your obliques.

A

POSITION
Sit on top of an exercise ball and place your feet flat on the floor. Slowly slide forward, rolling the bottom half of your glutes off the ball, until your lower back is centered atop the ball.

POSITION
Place your hands lightly behind your head to support it.

POSITION
Space your feet about 2 feet apart for better balance.

[FASTFACT]

Holding your breath during the rep not only better stabilizes your body but generates a little more force to complete the contraction. Exhale only at the top of the rep. Rep to just one side first or alternate reps.

FORM
Don't pull on your head in an effort to go higher.

MAKE IT HARDER

Hold a weight plate behind your head — besides increasing resistance, it keeps your hands and arms in place. That makes it harder to cheat by flapping your elbows across your body.

MOVEMENT
Crunch forward by squeezing your abs, rotating one elbow toward the opposite knee on the way up. Return to the start and stretch your abs fully.

BREATH
Exhale as you reach the top position.

[TIP43]

It's critical not to simply flap your elbow across your body — you need to fully rotate your torso and bring your arm and shoulder as a unit toward your opposite-side knee.

FORM
Consciously push your lower back into the ball, which enables you to go higher at the top.

B

SKILL
LEVEL

2

Crossover Tuck Crunch

One of the many variations of the standard crunch, this exercise works all three major areas of your midsection.

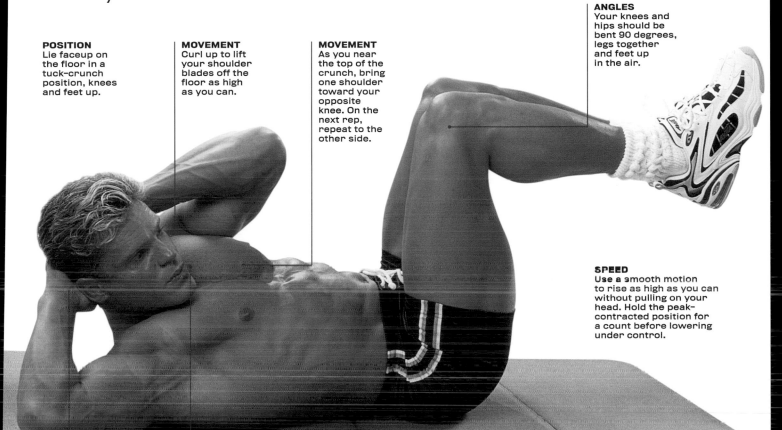

ANGLES
Your knees and hips should be bent 90 degrees, legs together and feet up in the air.

POSITION
Lie faceup on the floor in a tuck-crunch position, knees and feet up.

MOVEMENT
Curl up to lift your shoulder blades off the floor as high as you can.

MOVEMENT
As you near the top of the crunch, bring one shoulder toward your opposite knee. On the next rep, repeat to the other side.

SPEED
Use a smooth motion to rise as high as you can without pulling on your head. Hold the peak-contracted position for a count before lowering under control.

POSITION
Cup your hands lightly behind your head to support it.

BREATH
Exhale at the top of the movement.

[FASTFACT]

Holding your feet in the air forces your lower abs to contract. This contraction is isometric, however, and shouldn't take the place of a dynamic lower-ab movement.

MAKE IT HARDER

Fully extend your legs straight above you and split your feet about 2 feet apart. Reach with your hands for alternate feet, and try to go higher on each rep without using any body english.

[TIP44]

On the way down, don't allow your head or shoulders to fully touch the floor to maintain tension on your abs. Your feet shouldn't return to the floor until your set is complete.

[COMBOS]

V-Up

A more complex move that works both the upper and lower abs through a dynamic range of motion.

POSITION
Lie on the floor, legs straight and arms close by your sides. Bring your shoulders a few inches off the floor while simultaneously bringing your feet up to the same height.

FORM
Keep your head neutrally aligned with your spine.

POSITION
Your hands should be elevated about 10 inches off the floor.

A

MOVEMENT
Crunch up with your upper body, going as high as you can.

BREATH
Exhale as you reach the top position.

MOVEMENT
Reach up to touch your toes while simultaneously raising your legs as high as you can.

SPEED
Make sure the motion is smooth and continuous; don't jerk your body or lose control of the negative rep.

B

[FASTFACT]

Balancing your body is important here. Practice balancing on just your glutes, lowering your hands to track just off the floor to start. Or sit on a flat bench and lightly grasp its edges behind your hips.

12

After you can do more than **12 reps**, make the movement more challenging by slowing your rep speed or taking a shorter rest period.

[TIP45]

If the standard V-Up is too difficult, try pulling your knees into your chest and crunching up at the same time, reaching with your hands to the outsides of your feet.

SKILL LEVEL
3

Exercise-Ball Transfer Crunch
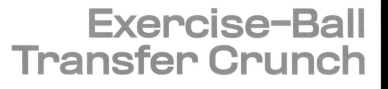

POSITION
Lie faceup on the floor, placing the ball between your ankles and keeping it there by lightly pressing your legs together. Raise the ball off the floor about 6 inches.

A

POSITION
Extend your arms straight overhead.

MOVEMENT
Raise your legs straight up, bringing the ball over your midsection.

To blast both the upper- and lower-ab regions, rise as high as you can to pass the exercise ball back and forth between your hands and feet.

MOVEMENT
At the same time, crunch up to move your hands into position to meet the ball. Transfer the ball to your hands.

BREATH
Exhale at the top.

FORM
As your upper body descends, allow your arms to return overhead, ball in hands, but don't let it touch the floor. Reverse the motion as you transfer the ball back to your feet in the top position.

B

MOVEMENT
Lower your legs back to the 0-inch point.

C

FORM
Keep your head neutrally aligned throughout the rep; your chin should never press against your chest.

[FASTFACT]
Your adductor and hip flexor muscles are highly recruited during this move. To boost the work in your lower abs, make sure you curl the lower portion of your glutes up off the floor.

MAKE IT HARDER
As your core strength increases, begin using medicine balls of different circumferences and weights. When you change up these variables, slow your rep speed until you get the feel of the motion.

[TIP46]
This exercise is designed to maintain constant tension on the abs. Don't allow your feet, hands or the ball to rest on the floor at any point during the movement.

COMBOS

Reverse Oblique Crunch

Similar to the reverse crunch, this move trains your lower abs while adding some side-to-side work for your obliques.

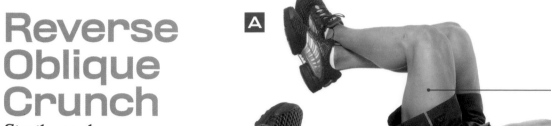

A

POSITION
Get into the tuck-crunch position, knees and hips bent about 90 degrees, feet up and thighs perpendicular to the floor. Cross your ankles.

POSITION
Lie faceup on the floor.

POSITION
Place your hands lightly behind your head to support it and maintain alignment.

MOVEMENT
Use your lower abs to roll your pelvis upward and lift your glutes off the floor.

MOVEMENT
As your knees come toward your chest, point them in the direction of one shoulder, then return under control and repeat to the opposite side.

BREATH
Exhale at the top of the movement.

SPEED
Use a smooth, controlled speed on both the positive and negative portions of the rep.

FORM
Your glutes should come off the mat at the top of each rep.

B

[FASTFACT]

To work your lower abs, you need to get the lower portion of your glutes off the mat. Crunch your sides hard to bring your knees high over your chest and activate your obliques.

MAKE IT HARDER

Hold a lightweight dumbbell or medicine ball between your feet, or perform the exercise on an incline bench. In either case, pay close attention to controlling the negative portion of the rep.

[TIP47]

Range of motion is important in this exercise, so contract your obliques hard and curl your glutes as high off the mat as possible to achieve the best results.

SKILL
LEVEL

3

Decline-Bench Twisting Crunch

Add a twist to the standard decline crunch for an excellent upper-ab and obliques move.

POSITION
Place your hands lightly behind your head to support it.

MOVEMENT
Stop about two-thirds of the way down to stretch your abs before going into the next rep.

POSITION
Secure your feet under the ankle pads.

A

MOVEMENT
Twist as you're coming up to bring one elbow toward your opposite knee. Alternate sides for reps.

FORM
Your hip flexors are highly activated during this movement, so try not to squeeze your quads to pull through your legs.

FORM
Round your back to increase your abdominal contraction as you rise.

MOVEMENT
Contract your abs to curl up to a point where you're just past perpendicular to the bench.

B

[FASTFACT]
You can adjust the angle of the decline bench to adapt this movement to your own personal training level — anywhere from beginner to advanced.

MAKE IT HARDER
Try alternating these twisting reps for your obliques with straight up-and-down reps for your upper abs to turn this into an advanced exercise.

[TIP48]
Start with a steep decline and, as your abs become fatigued, lower the angle to do more sets. That way you can get a thorough upper-ab workout with one piece of equipment.

COMBOS

SKILL LEVEL

3

Cycling With Ball

Though it takes a bit of coordination, this exercise is good for hitting all your major midsection muscles and can be done for high reps to really burn them out.

FORM
Keep your head neutrally aligned and facing forward.

A

POSITION
Hold a medicine ball over your chest or midsection.

POSITION
Begin in the jackknife position (similar to the V-up) with your upper body and legs in the air, balancing on your glutes.

BREATH
Exhale as you reach the endpoint in the range of motion.

MOVEMENT
As you extend one leg, flex the other to bring your knee toward your body.

MOVEMENT
Simultaneously rotate your torso to bring the ball toward that knee. Reverse motions and shift the ball to the other side to meet the opposite knee.

SPEED
Keep the motion smooth and continuous.

B

[FASTFACT]

During this exercise, your upper abs undergo a strong isometric contraction to hold your torso in place while your obliques and lower abs do the majority of the active work.

MAKE IT HARDER

Try using a heavier medicine ball or ankle weights to add resistance. You could also gauge your sets by time instead of reps, increasing the length of your intervals by several seconds on each rep.

[TIP49]

Don't just move your arms across your body to meet the opposite knee — actually rotate your torso as your hands and the ball stay in the same relative position.

COMBOS

Double-Crunch Leg Raise

SKILL LEVEL

3

A

POSITION
Extend your legs and hold your heels about 6 inches off the floor.

POSITION
Lie faceup on the floor.

POSITION
Lightly support your head with your hands, just off the floor to start.

FORM
Keep your feet together throughout the motion.

FORM
Don't pull on your head in an effort to go higher.

MOVEMENT
Bring your knees in toward your chest. At the same time, lift the lower portion of your glutes off the floor.

BREATH
Exhale at the point of peak contraction at the top of the movement.

MOVEMENT
Curl your upper body as high as it can go, trying to lift your shoulder blades off the floor.

This intermediate-level bodyweight movement works both ends of your rectus abdominis with a greater range of motion.

B

COMBOS

[FASTFACT]

This movement requires a great deal of balance and coordination, and when it's performed correctly, you don't have any opportunity to rest between reps.

MAKE IT HARDER

Extend your arms overhead and cross your palms, similar to the way you'd perform an arms-overhead crunch. Or try carefully holding a small dumbbell or weight plate behind your head.

[TIP 50]

Try kicking your legs all the way out. Don't allow them to touch the floor or kick them too high, both of which are cheating — they should hover a few inches off the floor at the bottom.

SKILL
LEVEL

4

Decline Twisting Crunch With Medicine Ball

A

MOVEMENT
Stop about two-thirds of the way down to stretch your abs before going into the next rep.

When decline twisting crunches become too easy, hold a medicine ball to add resistance and shape up your upper abs and obliques.

POSITION
Hold a medicine ball over your midsection and keep it in the same relative position as you twist.

POSITION
Secure your feet under the rollers.

MOVEMENT
Contract your abs to curl up to a point where you're just past perpendicular to the bench.

FORM
Round your back to increase your abdominal contraction as you rise.

FORM
Twist as you crunch up, aiming one shoulder toward the opposite knee and carrying the ball with you. Alternate sides every rep.

FORM
Your hip flexors are highly activated during this movement, so try not to squeeze your quads to pull through your legs.

B

[FASTFACT]

There are a couple of ways to modify the difficulty level of this exercise. More advanced trainees can adjust the angle of decline on the bench or increase the weight of the ball.

MAKE IT HARDER

Alternate these twisting reps, which emphasize your obliques, with straight up-and-down reps, which target your upper abs, to transform this exercise into a highly advanced move.

[TIP51]

Don't just move the ball to one side as you rise — turn your shoulder toward your opposite side, rotating your torso and the ball. This is a far superior way to work your obliques.

SKILL
LEVEL

4

Hanging Knee Raise to Side

It may look like you're just monkeying around, but this exercise requires strength, focus and coordination.

A

GRIP
Grasp the bar with an overhand grip, your hands a comfortable distance apart.

MOVEMENT
Don't swing your legs behind you at the bottom of the rep to gather momentum for the next rep. Come to a full stop or have a partner slow your momentum after each rep.

POSITION
Allow your body to hang freely, arms fully extended.

POSITION
Put a slight bend in your hips at the bottom.

POSITION
Bend your knees and lock them in this position for the entire set.

BREATH
Exhale as you reach the top position.

FORM
Try to bring your top knee as high as possible while keeping your legs and feet together.

MOVEMENT
Slowly lift your knees as high as you can to one side. Think of curling your spine from the bottom up, not simply lifting your knees.

SPEED
Use a controlled motion — swinging your body robs your muscles of the workload.

B

[FASTFACT]

Most hanging exercises like this one can also be done on a vertical bench, which doesn't require you to hold onto a bar and provides some back support to reduce body swing.

MAKE IT HARDER
It's difficult to add extra weight on this move. Instead, increase the angle in your knees to lengthen the lever or do oblique crunches on a cable apparatus, although those hit your upper, not lower, abs.

[TIP52]

Use ab straps if your grip starts to give out before your abs do in order to take your sets to failure. Be sure to perform the same number of reps on both sides.

[COMBOS]

Oblique Cable Crunch

This effective upper-ab and obliques move allows for varying levels of resistance based on your ability.

FORM
Grasp a rope handle attached to a high-pulley cable. Bend your arms to about 90 degrees and hold your hands near your forehead. Lock your arms in this position.

ANGLES
Kneel about 2 feet from the apparatus and angle your body about 45 degrees to it. Bend forward at the hips about 30 degrees to start.

MOVEMENT
Simultaneously crunch down and twist away from the machine, moving one elbow toward the opposite knee. Do all reps for one side first, then reposition your body for the other side's reps.

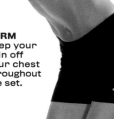

POSITION
Your back should be straight at the top, head neutrally aligned.

FORM
Keep your chin off your chest throughout the set.

BREATH
Exhale at the bottom of the rep.

FORM
Your head should follow your hands and torso.

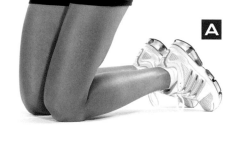

A

FORM
Keep your arms locked in position to prevent them from assisting in the movement.

B

FORM
Don't allow your glutes to sit back as you complete the movement.

SPEED
Use a forceful but smooth speed on the positive motion and control the negative to more thoroughly work your midsection.

[FASTFACT]

The standing version allows you to better emphasize your obliques; here, you simultaneously crunch and twist, so you're working both your upper abs and obliques.

MAKE IT HARDER
Try alternating reps to each side for your obliques with straight up-and-down reps for your upper abs to turn this into an advanced exercise. Just add weight when you're ready for more resistance.

[TIP53]

Think about rounding your back as you crunch down and to the side. Hold the peak contraction for a count, squeezing both your abs and obliques. Train both sides.

Ab Wheel

This ab contraption actually works and it's definitely harder than it looks, activating your core, lats and hip flexors as well as your abs.

SETUP
Use a smooth surface that won't cause the wheel to snag but one soft enough to not hurt your knees.

POSITION
Kneel on the floor with your feet behind you, knees just slightly apart. Bend over at the waist so your torso is slightly inclined.

POSITION
Keep your head neutrally aligned throughout.

POSITION
Hold the wheel about 6 inches in front of your knees so that your arms hang straight down, elbows bent slightly.

GRIP
Take firm hold of the wheel's handles.

SKILL LEVEL
4

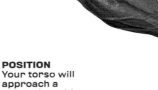

A

MOVEMENT
Slowly roll the wheel straight out in front of you, but don't go too far. Contract your abs to bring yourself up, and try to round your back as if you were a cat stretching its back.

FORM
Keep your head neutrally aligned.

BREATH
Don't exhale until you get back to the top position.

SPEED
Make the motion smooth and controlled.

POSITION
Your torso will approach a point where it's almost level with the floor.

B

[FASTFACT]
Do the most difficult moves in your workout first when your abs are fresh. Finish up with slightly easier exercises to continue challenging your fatiguing abs.

MAKE IT HARDER
Try rolling the wheel farther away from your body, which forces your body closer to the floor, dramatically increasing the level of difficulty of this exercise.

[TIP54]
Start with a small range of motion and slowly increase how far the wheel travels from your body till you get the hang of the move and your ab strength increases.

COMBOS

SKILL LEVEL

4

Barbell Ab Roll

This challenging exercise is a great functional movement for building overall core strength.

SETUP
Load a barbell with 25-, 35- or 45-pound circular plates and set it on the floor. Heavier weights raise your hand position slightly higher off the floor and are more difficult to move across the floor.

A

POSITION
Stand behind the barbell in a hip-width stance. Bend over and grasp the bar with a shoulder-width grip, rounding your lower back.

FORM
Be sure to keep your shoulders over your hands at all times.

POSITION
Rise up onto your toes.

BREATH
Exhale as you reach the extended position.

SPEED
Make the motion smooth and continuous.

MOVEMENT
Slowly roll the barbell forward until your body is fully extended (or as far as you can go). Concentrate on slowly lengthening your abs.

MOVEMENT
Drive your hips toward the ceiling as you roll the barbell back toward your feet.

B

[FASTFACT]

Training your torso in a vertical position, as seen here, is ideal for building strength for standing exercises like squats, deadlifts, shoulder presses and curls.

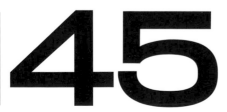

45 Instead of using smaller plates (quarters), try the **35s or 45s** for increased resistance.

[TIP55]

When you first begin performing this exercise, don't roll the bar out very far. As you get the hang of the movement, try to increase the distance the barbell travels on the floor.

[COMBOS]

SKILL
LEVEL

5

Windshield Wiper

As impressive to watch as it is difficult to perform, this exercise requires not only strong abs but good flexibility.

POSITION
Grasp a pull-up bar with an overhand grip. Take a deep breath and contract your abs to raise your legs all the way up — ankles to your forehead — with a slight bend in your knees. Your body should look like a "V."

A

FORM
Your arms should be nearly straight.

BREATH
Exhale as you bring your legs back up to the top position on each rep.

FORM
Your hips should be flexed in the "V" position for the entire set.

CAUTION
For safety, have a spotter on hand to help you get into position the first few times you do this move.

MOVEMENT
Slowly move your legs to the left of your body about 90 degrees, then repeat to the right side.

FORM
Your upper body should stay in the same relative position throughout the movement.

SPEED
Keep this movement carefully controlled.

B

[FASTFACT]
During this exercise, your upper abs undergo a strong isometric contraction, while your lower abs do a substantial amount of work and your obliques are trained hard.

MAKE IT HARDER
Alternate reps of the windshield wiper with hanging leg raises in which you bring your ankles all the way up to your forehead. Get it right and you qualify for the next ab-infomercial gig.

[TIP56]
Work through a small range of motion until you get the hang of this exercise. Also, work on hamstring flexibility if you have difficulty bringing your ankles to your forehead.

COMBOS

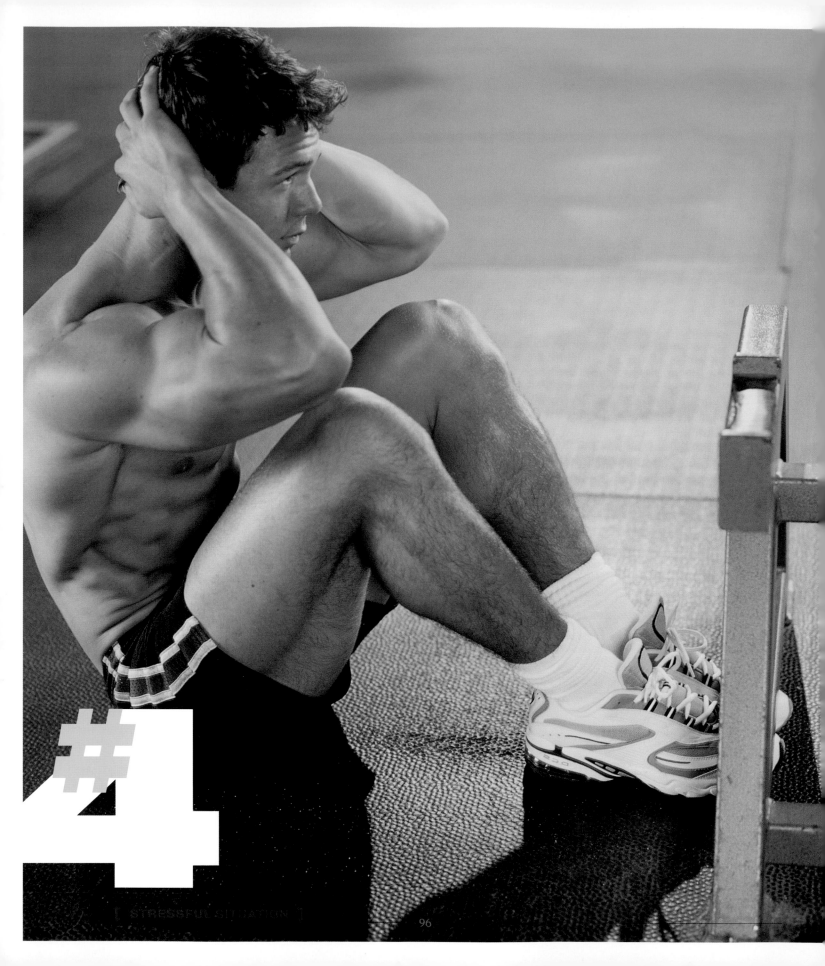

4

Four Worst Ab Exercises

IF YOU WANT RESULTS, TRADE IN THESE CLUNKERS FOR PROVEN AB MOVES

Let's face it: Ab exercises aren't easy. In fact, if done correctly, they can be downright brutal, inciting a muscle burn in your midsection rivaling the five-alarm jalapeño-and-chili-pepper burrito special at the local Taco Palace. Knowing that you want two things out of your ab workout — brevity and results — you'll want to be careful to choose exercises that are up to the task. With that in mind, we present the four worst ab exercises, along with some reasons why you shouldn't waste your time on these outdated moves.

4) Traditional Sit-Up

Ranking fourth is one that used to be a stalwart — back in the "prehistoric" days of lifting, at least. The traditional sit-up — where you lie on the floor, knees bent, and sit all the way up to bring your elbows to your knees — is an exercise you may have been doing since grade school. Yet the mere fact that your burly gym teacher prescribed it certainly doesn't make it right.

The sit-up does involve an ab contraction, but it also puts unwanted stress on the lower spine because of the extreme range of motion. According to Wendell P. Liemohn, PhD, professor of exercise science at the University of Tennessee, Knoxville, the psoas magnus muscle in the lower back, which is one of the muscles that brings the thighs and pelvis together, is very active in the sit-up. "The psoas muscle is so positioned that it can place extreme compressive forces on the spine, [specifically the] intervertebral discs," he explains. Since the psoas is intricately wrapped around the spine, it creates compressional forces on the intervertebral discs when contracted. In addition, locking your feet under a pad or bar increases hip flexor involvement, allowing you to do the movement in a greater range of motion but doing little for the abdominals.

Instead of a sit-up, try a crunch, which involves a very small range of motion, thus hitting the abs without putting your low back at risk by activating the psoas.

3) Crossover Sit-Up

In this sit-up variation, you bring your left elbow to your right knee and vice versa. The theory is that it works the oblique muscles, which run along the sides of the rectus abdominis. The reality is that this type of move increases spinal compression. Also, like the sit-up, coming all the way up relies on the hip flexors and psoas.

Although a standard crunch was a good replacement for the sit-up, a crunch with a twist is a distant second to replace a crossover sit-up, if only because you have a few more direct

#2

[NOT GOOD FOR THE SPINE]

QUICKTIP

>> The broomstick twist involves rotation in the lower-back region that's not good for your spine. Also, the exercise is powered by momentum rather than muscle. Don't waste your time on this move.

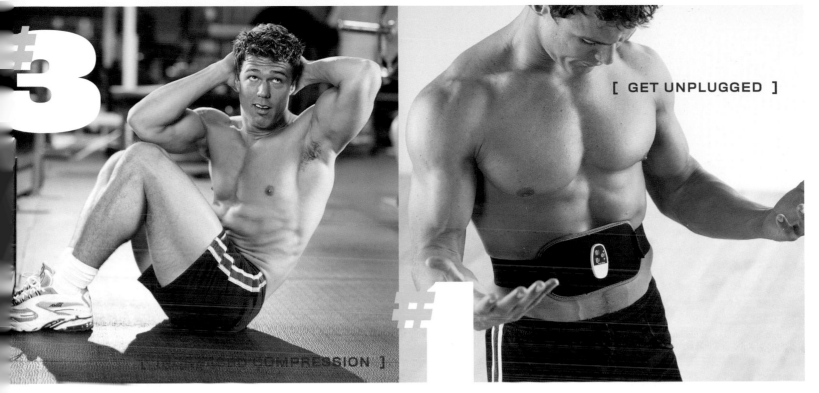

3

[COMPRESSION]

1

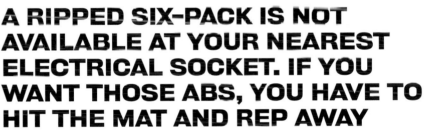

A RIPPED SIX-PACK IS NOT AVAILABLE AT YOUR NEAREST ELECTRICAL SOCKET. IF YOU WANT THOSE ABS, YOU HAVE TO HIT THE MAT AND REP AWAY

choices for your obliques. Try a hanging knee raise to the side instead, bringing your hip toward your shoulder on one side and then the other for reps, or a lying oblique crunch, in which you position your legs to the side, one on top of the other.

2) Broomstick Twist

Is there anything more pathetic than the lonely guy in the corner of the gym, doing hundreds of reps of standing twists while holding a pole across his shoulders? It's probably the ultimate example of the spot-reduction myth — but no, just because you're moving right in that area where your love handles are doesn't mean they're melting away with every twist.

The broomstick twist is fallible on many levels. First, it involves rotation in the lower-back region that, as mentioned, is not good for the spine. Second, the exercise is powered by momentum rather than muscle. Slow and conscious contraction of the obliques is far better. And last, it's just not cool to be

known as "that broomstick twist dude" at the gym.

A good replacement? A crunch, a hanging knee raise, a reverse crunch, a cable crunch, a hanging knee raise to the side...save the exercises on this list, almost anything is a preferred alternative to the broomstick twist. To get rid of those love handles, start doing your cardio and keep an eye on your diet.

1) EMS Devices

If you've ever been wide awake at 3 in the morning with a remote control in one hand and a protein shake in the other, you've seen the infomercials for electrical muscle-stimulation devices, which promise perfect abs without working out. Yep, just strap on the electrodes and a current will do the work for you while you sit in the recliner.

Unfortunately, the old adage is true: You only get out what you put in. A ripped six-pack isn't available at your nearest electrical socket. If you want those abs, you have to hit the mat and start repping. Now get to it!

CHAPTER FOUR

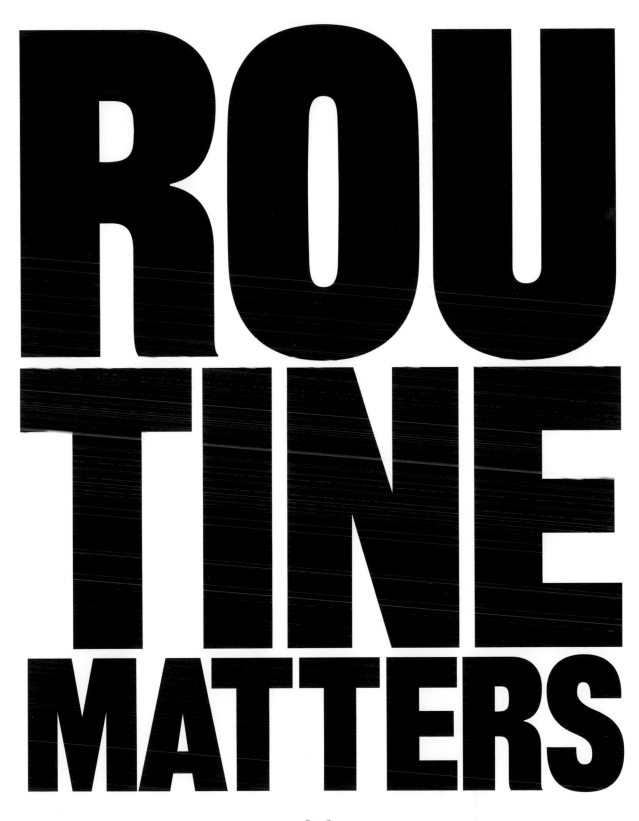

ROU
TINE
MATTERS

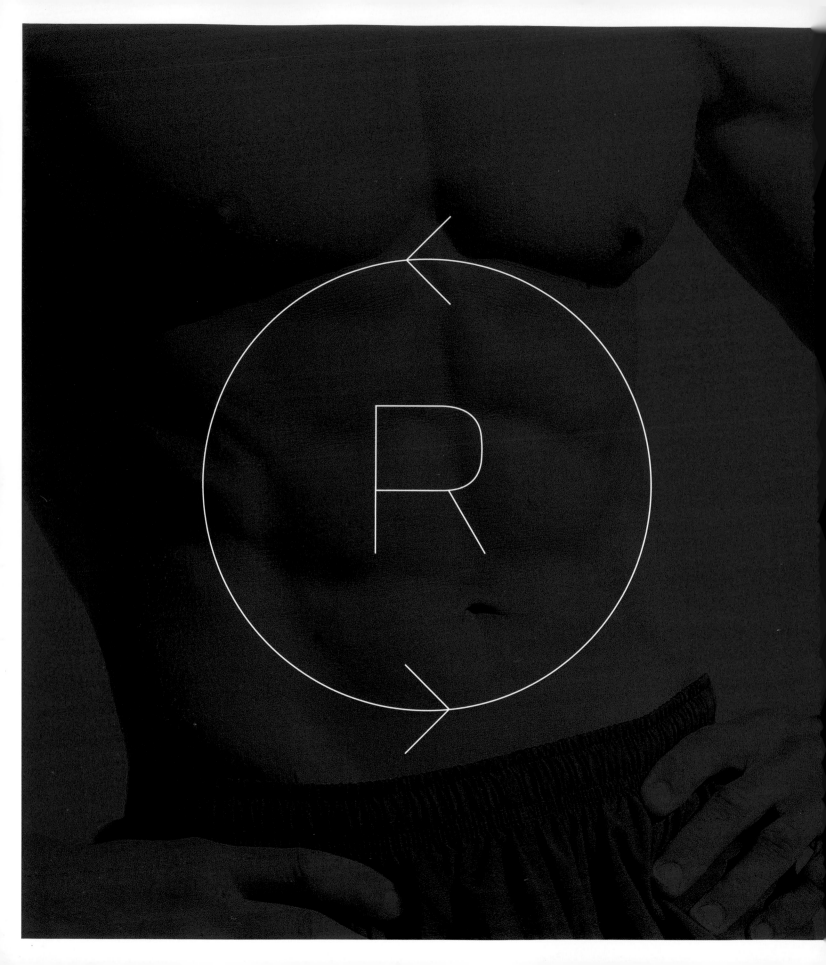

Building a Better Routine

HERE ARE THE ESSENTIAL TIPS YOU NEED TO CREATE A ROCK-HARD AB WORKOUT

Eat right and do crunches. Maybe twists...leg raises...crossovers...sit-ups. Heck, why not just do 30 minutes of various ab exercises? *Grooaan!* ¶ That's one way to train your abs, though it's not a particularly smart one. Sure, you can train your abs in countless fashions, combining an assortment of moves, sets and reps, but some strategies are far superior to others. Here, we'll explain the most important considerations in putting together an effective ab workout, one that'll help you realize your goal of a chiseled six-pack.

1) Your Goals Dictate Your Training Approach

Unlike most major muscles, the abs are almost always in a state of contraction as they work to maintain good posture (both in daily activities and in the gym) and hold in the internal organs. That's why they have a greater endurance component than most muscle groups, which may explain why they're often trained more frequently with higher repetitions.

If you want a strong, well-toned midsection, perform about 20 reps per set with moderate resistance. (One important reminder: Because you can't spot-reduce, don't expect to build definition — that is, an extreme degree of leanness — in your abs this way.) If your goal is to develop thicker abs with noticeable peaks and valleys, use a traditional regimen of heavy resistance with lower reps. Select an exercise or a resistance that allows you to do 10–12 repetitions, which is slightly higher than for other bodyparts. The last several reps should be difficult to complete and cause a burning sensation in the ab muscles.

One important point that affects how many reps you do relates to how hard you "crunch" your abs at the top of each movement. Unless your abs are extremely tired, you should probably get at least 10 reps. If you can do more than 25–30, you probably aren't putting enough intensity into each rep. Slow down and really focus on contracting your abs at the top of each rep.

2) Target Particular Areas of the Midsection

Although the rectus abdominis is a single muscle, you can work it from different angles to better target particular areas, somewhat similar to how incline presses emphasize your upper chest. Though you can never truly isolate the upper-ab region from the lower, particular exercises more effectively work one or the other. The difference isn't dramatic, but it is enough to suggest doing a variety of ab movements.

In general, stabilizing your upper torso and raising your pelvis (and feet) will work the lower-ab region more strongly, while curling your shoulder blades and ribcage toward your stabilized pelvis and lower body works the upper abs more strongly. A third portion of a good ab workout is often dedicated to the external obliques. They're typically involved in movements in which one shoulder crosses the body toward the opposite knee.

Start Your Routine With Lower Abs

Though this technique is still subject to debate, working the lower-abdominal region first is a smart idea because it's generally weaker, requires more coordinated movement patterns and must be stabilized by the stronger obliques and upper-ab area. The lower-ab region's weakness is due in part to less-frequent training but more so to the involvement of the hip flexors that assist with many lower-abdominal movements. In addition, the obliques and upper abs need to stabilize and immobilize the upper abs during lower-ab training, so they must be fresh and strong to ensure that you can maintain proper form (which wouldn't happen if you did upper abs first). Good form for lower-ab movements means minimal hip-flexor movement and maximal contraction of the lower-abdominal region.

With numerous lower-ab exercises to choose from, it's difficult to make a case for a single "best" exercise to start with. Given your goals and ability level, select an exercise that induces muscle fatigue at your target rep range. A beginner who wants to build thicker abs probably wouldn't choose the same exercise as a beginner who wants to build muscular endurance but little thickness; the former would opt for a more difficult exercise with greater resistance for fewer reps (see "Lower-Ab Exercises" in chart below). Experiment with various movements to determine which feel best and challenge you. Do at least two sets to focus on each region of the abs, remembering that truly intense repetitions will generate better results than endless low-intensity reps. As you advance, you can add more exercises and sets.

If you perform more than one movement that targets a particular region, start with the most difficult one. A muscle is always stronger on the first exercise than on subsequent moves, so you wouldn't want to do your hardest movement last. For example, reverse crunches on a flat bench are typically easier than hanging leg raises, so do the leg raises first if you include both in your lower-ab workout.

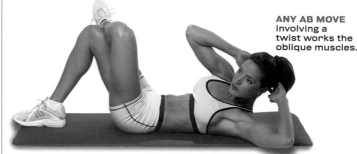

ANY AB MOVE involving a twist works the oblique muscles.

Hit the Obliques Next

If you train your midsection from weakest to strongest, next in line is generally the obliques. As with other areas of the midsection, use a critical eye when deciding if you want to thicken your obliques by using heavy resistance; this can make you appear blockier in the middle and works against a nicely shaped V-taper.

Oblique exercises also range in difficulty, and many of them are combination movements in which you do a crunch for upper abs with a twist for obliques (see "Oblique Exercises" in chart below). Again, try different ones to see which are most effective at inducing muscle fatigue in your target rep range.

Finish Off With Upper Abs

After you hit the lower abs and obliques, work your upper-ab region; the most effective exercises to do so are crunches. Here, your feet are stabilized and

Sample Exercises for a Six-Pack

BEGINNER	INTERMEDIATE	ADVANCED
LOWER-AB EXERCISES Pelvic Tilt, Reverse Crunch, Seated Knee-Up	**LOWER-AB EXERCISES** Vertical-Bench Knee Raise, Hanging Knee Raise, Hip Thrust	**LOWER-AB EXERCISES** Lower-Ab Machine, Partner-Assisted Leg Raise, Vertical-Bench Leg Raise, Hanging Leg Raise
OBLIQUE EXERCISES Twist, Side Jackknife, Oblique Crunch	**OBLIQUE EXERCISES** Cross-Body Crunch, Medicine-Ball Twist, Oblique Crunch, Side Bend	**OBLIQUE EXERCISES** Side Leg Raise, Cable Woodchop
UPPER-AB EXERCISES Curl-Up (hands outstretched toward feet), Crunch (hands crossed over chest), Supported Crunch, Butterfly Crunch	**UPPER-AB EXERCISES** Hands-Overhead Crunch, Straight-Leg Crunch, Exercise-Ball Crunch, Tuck Crunch	**UPPER-AB EXERCISES** Machine Crunch, Cable Crunch, Medicine-Ball Crunch, Decline-Bench Crunch

A MUSCLE IS ALWAYS WEAKER ON SUBSEQUENT EXERCISES, SO DO YOUR MOST DIFFICULT MOVEMENT FIRST RATHER THAN LAST IN YOUR ROUTINE.

you curl your upper torso toward your pelvis. The actual range of motion, as in many ab exercises, is fairly small but very effective if you use a controlled pace and flex your abs hard at the top of each crunch. Don't come all the way to the floor at the bottom of the rep, which would allow you to rest between reps. (See "Upper-Ab Exercises" in chart on previous page.)

Remember, you can usually make an exercise more difficult by changing your hand and/or foot placement. Moving your hands from beside your knees to across your chest to behind your head to overhead increases the difficulty with each step. Moving your feet from a position flat on the floor to knees and hips bent 90 degrees to legs straight up also increases the level of difficulty. Use these various positions to continually challenge your abs into making incremental gains in strength and size.

If you do more than one upper-ab move, start with the most difficult exercise first.

Add Variety to Your Ab Routine

Once your lower-ab strength is on par with the rest of your midsection muscles, experiment with the order in which you train the three areas. Work the upper region first one day, obliques first the next and the lower region first in your last ab-training session of the week. Or you may try devoting a single training session to one particular area.

Another technique that works especially well for abs is performing tri-sets. Complete one set of a lower-ab move and follow it immediately with one set each for upper abs and obliques.

Remember, variety is the golden rule of progress. Don't do the same exercises and sets-and-reps combinations every workout.

When to Train Abs

The optimal time to train your abs comes down to personal preference. Your answers to these questions may affect when you choose to train them:

■ **Are your abs a lagging bodypart?** If so, prioritize your ab training to bring them up.

■ **If you train with weights, will you really be inclined to train abs after a strenuous weight workout?** If you're tired after a hard weightlifting session, you might have trouble dedicating sufficient energy to ab training. Instead, do your ab workout first. Keep in mind, though, that overly fatiguing your abs can detract from your subsequent training — the abs are stabilizer muscles that keep your body "tight" during many exercises. Starting off with abs on a day you work legs may not be such a good idea.

■ **Can you train abs on your nonlifting days?** Many abdominal exercises can be done at home, and a complete workout takes just a few minutes.

Training Frequency

You often hear individuals recommend training abs daily, but you wouldn't do that with any other muscle group, so why abs? The abs require direct stimulation and then rest in order to grow, and they can easily be overtrained.

That being said, the abs do seem to recover more quickly than larger muscle groups. A hard leg workout may have you limping around for several days, but your abs seem to be just fine within 48 hours. A good rule of thumb is that if your abs are still sore from a previous workout, they aren't ready to be trained again.

An effective training pattern might consist of three ab sessions each week, which allows for about 48 hours of recovery in between. Still, allow your recovery instincts to dictate when to train your abs again.

Last But Not Least: Diet & Cardio

Perhaps the most frustrating aspect of ab training is understanding that just because you work your abs hard doesn't mean you'll see visible results. A strong midsection isn't always ripped and well-defined. Certainly, good-looking abs don't come easy, especially if you haven't been blessed in the genetics department. If you tend to accumulate bodyfat around your midsection, developing that area takes more than exercise alone. Successful ab training is a precise combination of a healthy, well-rounded diet, a consistent cardiovascular routine and, of course, a comprehensive abdominal workout.

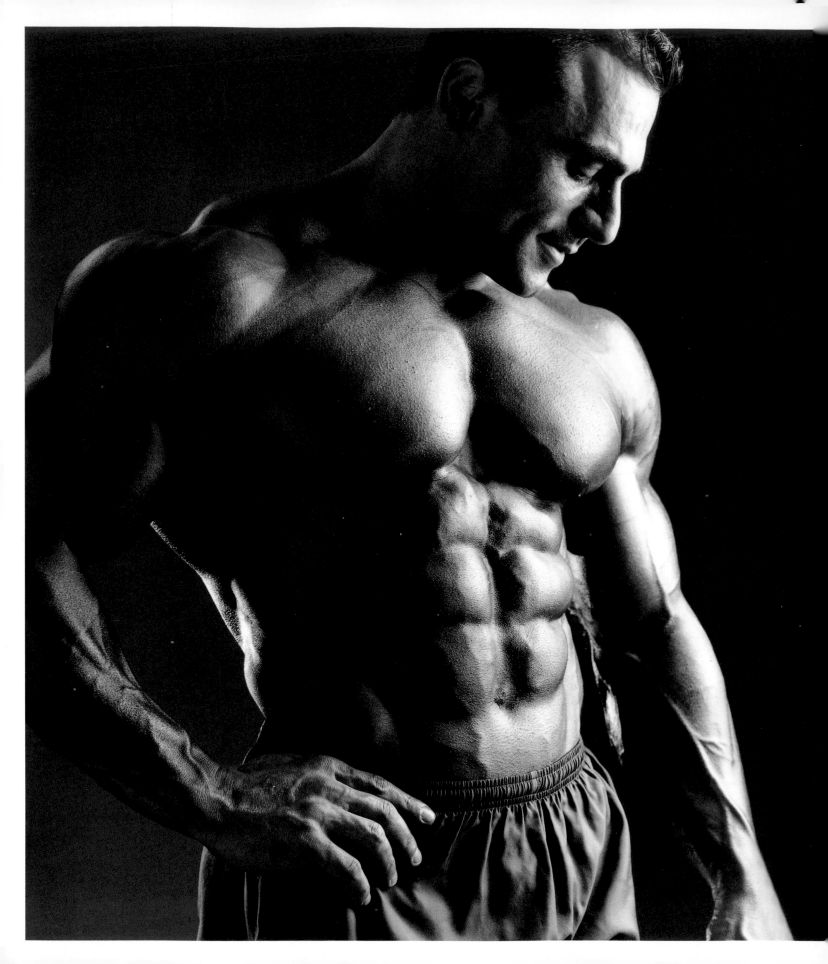

Seven Ways to a Six-Pack

SEVEN BODYBUILDER-TESTED WORKOUTS WILL TAKE YOU FROM FLAB TO ABS

Ah, the never-ending quest for abs. The eternal crusade for the Holy Grail of guts spawns crash diets, continuous crunches and incredulous ab-fomercial impulse buys on late-night TV. Unfortunately, there's no overnight way to procure that washboard stomach you long for. But with hard work, dedication and an unparalleled commitment to fitness, the following workouts will help set you on the path to Ab City. ❡ We consulted seven of the best bods in the biz, each with a unique style of training and novel insight into the mystery that is "the abs." Peruse their routines and ponder their advice, and use it to help you get a six-pack of your own.

[AHMAD HAIDAR]

"These days, I don't train abs specifically because I teach an abs class five days a week," explains Ahmad. "I do a half-hour class on continuous ab training with only 10–15 seconds rest between exercises." He'll choose 5–6 variations of crunches, a few oblique exercises and a couple of lower-ab leg raises for flavor. "High-rep ab training has always worked well for me, and I like that feeling of burning them out," says Ahmad. "For each exercise, we'll do 40–50 repetitions and will focus on using good form and complete range of motion on everything."

His favorite ab exercise is an oblique crunch with an added leg raise. "In this exercise, you raise both your upper and lower body at the same time and hold," he states. "That hits the entire length of your side and gives you a great burn!"

PERSONAL STATS

BIRTHDATE: April 10, 1968
HEIGHT: 5'7"
CONTEST WEIGHT: 220 pounds
IFBB pro competitor

EXERCISE	SETS	REPS
Crunch	5–6	40–50
Leg Raise	2–3	40–50
Oblique Crunch	2–3	20 each side
Side Leg Raise	2–3	20 each side
Bicycle Crunch	2–3	40–50

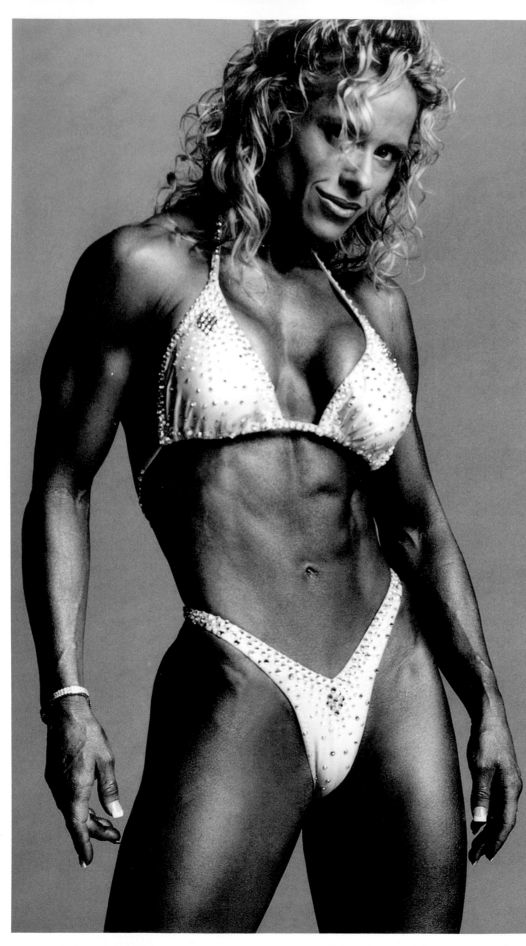

[MONICA BRANT]

Figure competitor and former fitness superstar Monica has some of the best-known abs in the industry. She keeps her midsection in top form by training it at least twice a week, using a high number of quality reps on each exercise in her routine. "Every rep of every set should be slow, controlled and executed with perfect form," she recommends.

Monica's ab regimen includes oblique crunches, weighted leg raises, hip thrusts and exercise-ball crunches. She enjoys a more challenging form of the leg raise: Lying on the floor, she stretches her arms out to her sides, then proceeds as usual with the move. By performing this exercise on the floor, she prevents her arms from providing any assistance and forces her abs to do all the work.

PERSONAL STATS
BIRTHDATE: Oct. 29, 1970
HEIGHT: 5'4"
CONTEST WEIGHT: 127 pounds
IFBB pro figure competitor

EXERCISE	SETS	REPS
Oblique Crunch	3	20–100 each side
Leg Raise (weighted)	3	20–100
Hip Thrust	3	20–50
Exercise-Ball Crunch	3	50–100

[RICHARD JONES]

As a police officer, it's Richard's job to look out for people's well-being. His concern extends into the gym as well: "The best way to start any ab movement is to make sure your body is in the right position and that everything is set up correctly," he advises. Once he's ready, he performs a hard-hitting workout that begins with four sets using an ab wheel to failure to really get a good burn going in his midsection. He proceeds to cable crunches, hanging leg raises and seated knee-ups, doing this six-pack-shredding routine every other day.

Ever mindful of safety, Richard emphasizes that each person should choose the ab moves that suit him or her best. "If you feel discomfort, don't do [the exercise]," he says. "It's not worth an injury."

PERSONAL STATS
BIRTHDATE: April 14, 1974
HEIGHT: 5'7"
CONTEST WEIGHT: 198 pounds
IFBB pro bodybuilder

EXERCISE	SETS	REPS
Ab Wheel	4	to failure
Cable Crunch	4	25
Hanging Leg Raise	4	20–25
Seated Knee-Up	4	10

To maintain his killer midsection, Stan takes an untraditional approach, training abs up to five times a week after every workout, which he feels works best for him. He believes in doing his ab exercises deliberately and with strict form, giving each rep his utmost attention. In turn, he doesn't require a high number of reps to achieve a good abdominal burn.

Stan's routine includes hanging leg raises, crunches of various types and V-ups on a bench. He finishes his workout with standing oblique cable crunches. He attaches a D-handle to the high pulley and then stands several feet away, his working side and arm facing the stack. With a palms-up grip, he pulls the handle toward his head. Keeping the same relative stance, Stan contracts his obliques to pull the handle downward, squeezing for 1–2 counts at the peak contraction. To put his obliques on stretch, he hyperextends slightly as he returns to the top.

PERSONAL STATS
BIRTHDATE: July 12, 1973
HEIGHT: 5'7"
CONTEST WEIGHT: 185 pounds
NPC amateur competitor

EXERCISE	SETS	REPS
Hanging Leg Raise	4	20
Crunch	4	20–30
V-Up on Bench	3	20–30
Standing Oblique Cable Crunch	3	20 each side

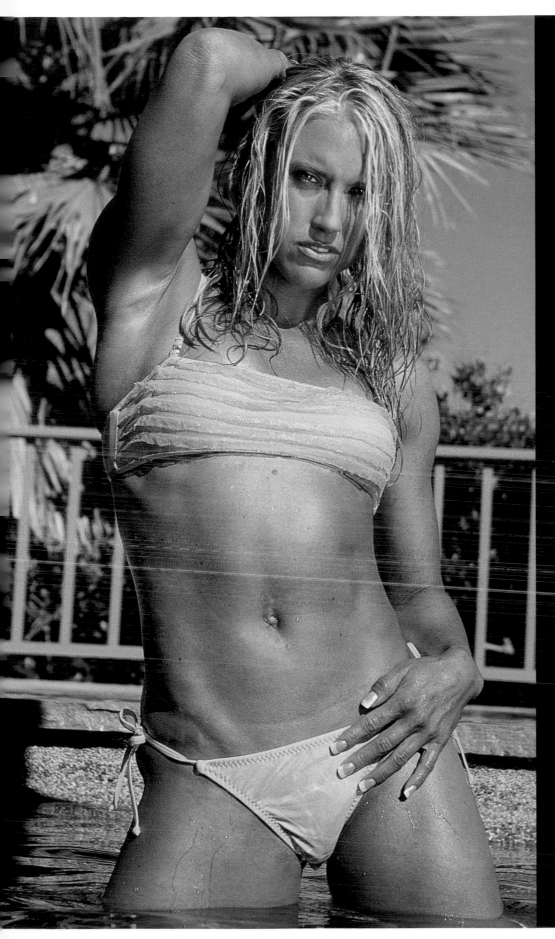

Instead of doing her ab work all at once, Beth mixes it into her routine for other bodyparts, performing ab exercises between sets. "I believe you should train abs just like any other muscle, so 8–10 reps is plenty for most exercises," she says. "I like to change variables with my ab training just like I do for other bodyparts, so I'll do things like negatives and supersets for my abs every other week or so."

Beth also performs an unusual variation of the hanging leg raise. "I like to do these on the Smith machine," she explains. "Set the bar at nose height and hang by your hands so that you look like you're sitting in the air. From here, lift your feet off the floor slightly so that you're hanging freely — that's your starting position. Then lift your knees up to your chest, pause and squeeze and slowly lower them back down to a position just above the floor. Then go right into the next repetition."

PERSONAL STATS
BIRTHDATE: Dec. 12
HEIGHT: 5'8"
CONTEST WEIGHT: 135 pounds
IFBB pro fitness competitor

EXERCISE	SETS	REPS
Medicine-Ball Decline Crunch	2–3	8–10
Hanging Leg Raise	3–4	10–12
Decline-Bench Reverse Crunch	3–4	10–15
Weighted Exercise-Ball Crunch	3–4	10

[VINCE GALANTI]

Vince trains his abs three times a week at the end of his workout. Because of a back injury he incurred as a teenager, he has to be careful about his choice of exercises. "I can't do regular leg raises on the floor or certain kinds of crunches," he explains. "So I've had to find exercises that don't aggravate my condition and play around with things so they don't hurt me."

Vince usually begins with reverse crunches to warm up his lower back and target the lower abs. "I hold a 4-pound medicine ball between my knees to add a little resistance," he says. "I do these slowly to focus on the muscle and avoid injury." His next exercise, one-arm medicine-ball crunches, involves balancing the same ball over his head with one arm and lifting his upper body off the floor slightly. "I typically superset these with exercise-ball crunches to really work the center of my abs and burn it out," he notes. Vince finishes with cable crunches and back extensions.

PERSONAL STATS
BIRTHDATE: April 18, 1967
HEIGHT: 5'7"
CONTEST WEIGHT: 198 pounds
NPC amateur competitor

EXERCISE	SETS	REPS
Medicine-Ball Reverse Crunch	3–4	10–15
One-Arm Medicine-Ball Crunch	3–4	20 each side
Exercise-Ball Crunch	3–4	30–40
Cable Crunch	3–4	15–25
Back Extension	3	20–30

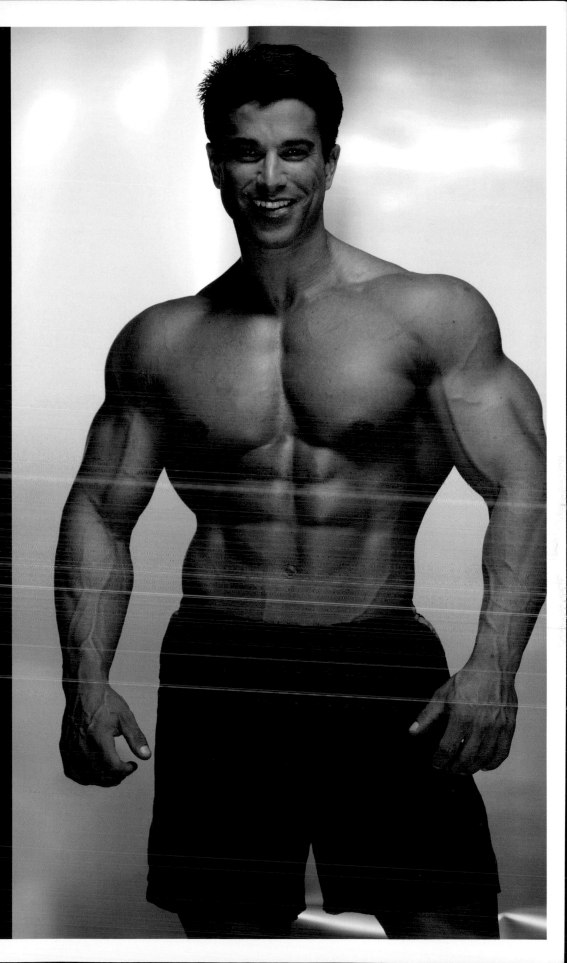

Sagi's rules for ab training are a little different than your average bodybuilder's because he doesn't really have any. "I like to mix things up to keep from getting bored," explains the eternally in-shape fitness model. And mix things up he does: Sagi alternates between working his abs before and after his routine, and he doesn't rely on a preset number of sets and reps to perform with each exercise. He prefers to think of them as guidelines, continuing with a move if he still has energy to do so.

Sagi suggests training abs no fewer than two times a week but no more often than every other day. "I've found that they're nearly impossible to overtrain," he says.

PERSONAL STATS

BIRTHDATE: July 30, 1971
HEIGHT: 5'8"
CONTEST WEIGHT: 195 pounds
Fitness model and former amateur bodybuilder

EXERCISE	SETS	REPS
Hanging Knee Raise	varies	varies
Lying Cable Crunch	varies	varies
Crossover Crunch	varies	varies

[CHAPTER FIVE]

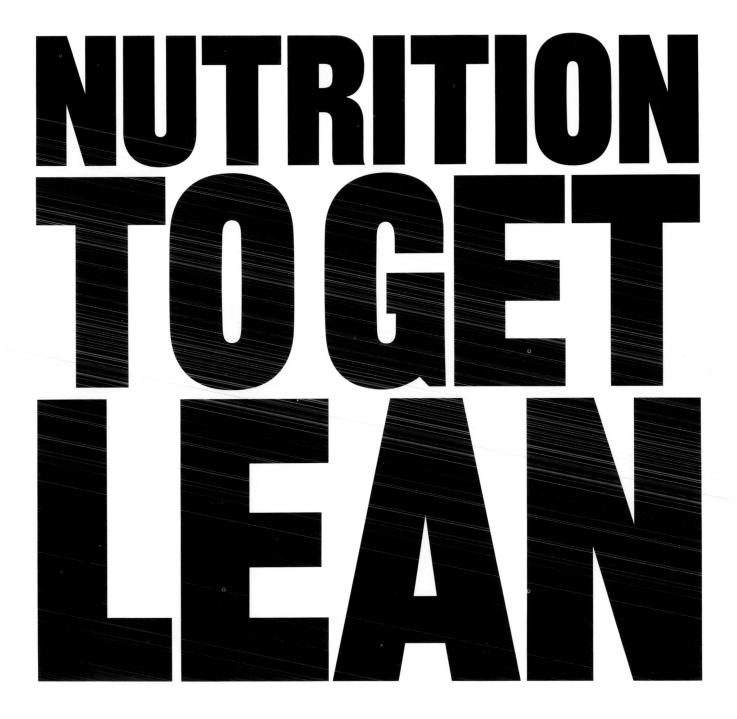

NUTRITION TO GET LEAN

Nutrition 101

USE THIS GUIDE TO CREATE THE ULTIMATE DIETARY PLAN FOR A LEANER, MORE ATHLETIC PHYSIQUE

Am I getting enough protein? Will carbs make me fat? How low should I go in my low-fat diet? What will give me more energy to train? What's the most important nutrient? ¶ The care and feeding of the human body seems complicated, but a few lessons in nutrition will simplify the process. Class, take note of your real protein needs, the importance of carbs for all active adults, the functions of fat, the fluid facts on hydration, and what and when to eat before and after you train. ¶ The final exam for Nutrition 101 is a take-home test: Put these lessons to work in your life for more energy, better health and a fitter body.

Protein The Muscle Builder

Strength athletes have routinely consumed diets extremely high in protein in hopes of increasing size, getting cut and gaining weight. Although protein performs important functions in the body as it relates to enzymes, hormones, immune-system antibodies and components of tissue, especially muscle, the effect of exercise on dietary protein requirements has been argued for the last 20 years.

The protein debate has fueled quite a bit of research, and it's now clear that regular exercise does in fact increase protein needs — good news for athletes who thought this was the case all along. Yet the interpretation of what the increase should be varies widely. The fact is that the typical American diet contains excess protein, so you can obtain sufficient protein without a lot of extra effort.

Do I Need a Protein Supplement?

Read food labels and use protein charts to track the number of grams of protein you eat each day. Do this for a few days to figure out your typical protein intake and adjust your diet accordingly. Remember, just because you lift weights doesn't mean you automatically need protein supplements. First determine your needs and then compare them with your average intake.

How Much Protein is Enough?

Consuming excess amounts of protein won't cause muscle growth. Truth is, muscle contraction through strength training is what stimulates muscle growth, and eating extra carbohydrate — stored as glycogen — fuels strength-training workouts. Without adequate glycogen, you can't optimally contract your muscles, which limits growth. Consuming carbs supports both glycogen and protein synthesis via your body's insulin response.

Research suggests that the protein intake for those who engage in regular strength-building exercise should be up to 1 gram per pound of bodyweight. Multiply your weight by the conversion factor of 0.4–1.0 (see chart at above left) to determine your daily protein needs.

THE PROTEIN DEBATE HAS FUELED QUITE A BIT OF RESEARCH, AND IT'S NOW CLEAR THAT REGULAR EXERCISE DOES IN FACT INCREASE PROTEIN NEEDS

PROTEININTAKE (based on activity)

ACTIVITY LEVEL	CONVERSION FACTOR
Sedentary individuals & sporadic exercisers	0.4 gram per pound bodyweight daily
Active exercisers	0.6–0.8 gram per pound bodyweight daily
Very active weightlifters & endurance athletes	1.0 gram per pound bodyweight daily

PROTEINCONTENT (of food groups)

FOOD GROUP	PROTEIN (G)	CALORIES
DAIRY — fat-free and low-fat 1 cup milk, ⅓ cup dry milk, ½ cup evaporated milk, ¾ cup yogurt	8	90–120
MEAT and meat substitutes 1 oz. lean meat, poultry, fish, shellfish, 2 egg whites, ½ cup cooked beans, 1 oz. low-fat cheese	7	35–55
STARCH 1 slice bread, ½ cup pasta, ⅓ cup rice, 1 small potato	3	80
VEGETABLES ½ cup cooked or 1 cup raw	2	25
FRUIT ½ cup juice or 1 piece raw	0	60

SOURCE: Wein, D., Economos, C. ENaO Pack: The Health Professionals' Guide to Sport Nutrition, 2000.

NUTRITIONVALUE (of various foods)

FOOD	CALORIES	PROTEIN (G)	CARBS (G)	FAT (G)	IRON (MG)	ZINC (MG)	POTASSIUM (MG)
1 cup fat-free milk	90	8	12	1	0.1	0.98	404
1 cup plain fat-free yogurt	110	12	16	0	16	149	497
1 oz. mozzarella (part skim)	79	8	1	5	0.07	0.89	27
1 oz. lean beef	62	9	0	3	0.98	1.55	87
1 oz. turkey	44	8.5	0	1	0.4	0.58	87
1 oz. tuna	33	7.3	0	1	0.43	0.22	67
2 egg whites	34	8	1	0	0.02	0.01	96
1 whole egg	74	6	1	5	0.72	0.55	80
½ cup garbanzo beans	134	7	23	2	2.4	1.2	239
2 Tbsp. peanut butter	190	8	7	16	0.54	0.81	232
1 slice whole-grain bread	64	2	12	1	0.87	0.26	46
½ cup pasta	100	3.5	20	1	0.98	0.37	38
½ cup brown rice	108	2.5	22.5	1	0.4	0.62	42
1 medium (7 oz.) potato	220	5	51	1	2.75	0.65	844
½ cup oatmeal (cooked)	70	3	12	1	4	0.6	89

Fat A Little Goes a Long Way

The word *fat* has been banned from some people's vocabulary, since extensive research supports the idea that diets high in total fat have been linked to obesity, heart disease, high blood cholesterol and some types of cancer. But fat also performs many important functions in the body, and many people completely ignore their body's requirement for healthy fats as they strive to eat a "fat-free" diet. You're wise to aim for 15%–25% of your daily total calories from fat; you don't need to cut your fat intake any lower than that.

Carbohydrates and proteins contain approximately 4 calories per gram, while fat contains 9. Therefore, cutting down on fat may help lower total calorie consumption, which can result in weight loss, but only if you don't increase portion sizes and number of servings. Be aware, however, that some reduced-fat or fat-free foods contain as many calories per serving as the higher-fat versions, so be sure to read labels.

YOU SHOULD EAT A FLAVORFUL, LOW-FAT DIET THAT'S BENEFICIAL TO YOUR HEALTH

Why Eat Fat?

Our bodies manufacture some fats and we also take in fats from the foods we eat. Fat enhances the flavor and texture of food, so meals with little or no fat don't provide the same satiety, or feeling of fullness. As a result, many people have given up on low-fat eating habits in exchange for higher-fat foods, which taste better. Bottom line: You should eat a flavorful, low-fat diet that's beneficial to your health.

What Are the Different Types of Fats?

When we consume fat, our bodies break it down to its smaller components, known as fatty acids. Depending on their chemical structure, these are called saturated, polyunsaturated or monounsaturated.

>> **Saturated fats,** the most common types of fat consumed in a typical diet, are found in animal foods such as meat, poultry and eggs, full-fat dairy products and tropical oils. Saturated fat is the type of fat most likely to travel through our arteries, depositing plaque and cholesterol, and raising low-density lipoprotein (LDL, or "bad") cholesterol. High intakes of saturated fats are linked to heart disease and some cancers, so experts recommend that your daily intake be less than 10% of your total calories.

>> **Polyunsaturated fats** (PUFAs) are found in foods like vegetable oils (safflower, sunflower and corn) and fatty fish. Although PUFAs provide linolenic and linoleic acid, both essential fatty acids that are necessary for health and

can't be made by the body, the daily recommended intake is less than 10% of total calories. Part of the omega-3 and omega-6 families, respectively, linolenic and linoleic acid serve as precursors to other crucial PUFAs. Some research suggests that omega-3 PUFAs may help prevent heart disease because they lower triglycerides and reduce blood clotting. They may also lower blood pressure and prevent irregular heartbeat.

>> **Monounsaturated fats** (MUFAs), found in foods such as vegetable oils (olive, peanut and canola), are the primary oil consumed in the heart-healthy Mediterranean diet. The daily recommended intake of MUFAs is 10% of total calories.

Decreasing your saturated fat intake and keeping your overall fat intake in perspective are equally important. Your diet shouldn't consist of too little or too much fat. Also keep in mind that foods lower in fat may not necessarily be lower in calories. In addition, caloric intake and physical activity have been overlooked in all the excitement regarding new fat-free and reduced-fat foods. Make a habit of reading labels to determine if a food has too much fat. Generally, a food should provide less than 3 grams of fat (27 fat calories) for every 100 calories it contains.

DAILY FAT INTAKE*

NUMBER OF CALORIES CONSUMED PER DAY	AIM FOR THIS MANY GRAMS OF FAT PER DAY
1,400	31–39
1,600	36–44
1,800	40–50
2,000	44–56
2,200	49–61
2,400	53–67
2,600	58–72
2,800	62–78
3,000	67–83

*NOTE: Calculations are based on 20%–25% of calories from fat.

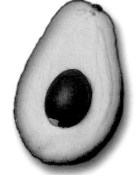

FAT FACT: THE AMAZING AVOCADO HAS HEALTHY MONOUNSATURATED FAT, VITAMINS, FIBER AND OTHER PROTECTIVE NUTRIENTS

FINDING FAT (in foods)

FOOD GROUP	FAT (G)	FOOD GROUP	FAT (G)
MEAT, FISH, POULTRY		BREADS, CEREALS	
Ground beef (4 oz.)	17	Shredded wheat (1 biscuit)	0
Lean ground beef (4 oz.)	10	White/brown rice (1 cup)	1
Ground turkey (4 oz.)	8	Pasta (1 cup plain)	1
Fried chicken breast	22	Oatmeal (1 cup cooked)	2
Baked skinless chicken breast (3 oz.)	4	White/wheat/rye bread (1 slice)	1
Bacon (2 slices)	14		
Roasted skinless turkey breast (3.5 oz.)	3	DAIRY PRODUCTS	
		Whole milk (1 cup)	8
Pork tenderloin (3 oz.)	5	2% milk (1 cup)	5
Tuna in oil (3 oz.)	7	Fat-free milk (1 cup)	0
Tuna in water (3 oz.)	1	Regular ice cream (¾ cup)	6
Baked haddock, cod (3.5 oz.)	2	Regular yogurt (1 cup)	7
		Low fat yogurt (1 cup)	3
FATS, OILS		Cottage cheese (4% fat — 1 cup)	8
Mayonnaise (1 Tbsp.)	11		
Salad dressing (1 Tbsp.)	8	American cheese (1 oz.)	9
Butter or margarine (1 Tbsp.)	12	Cheddar or blue cheese (1 oz.)	7
Oil (1 Tbsp.)	12	Cream cheese (1 oz.)	5

SOURCE: Wein, D., Economos, C. SNaC Pack: The Health Professionals' Guide to Sport Nutrition, 2000.

FUNCTIONS OF...

DIETARY FAT	FAT IN THE BODY
Concentrated source of energy, providing approximately 9 calories per gram	Provides fuel for daily activities and normal body metabolism
Provides a source of fat-soluble vitamins A, D, E and K	Provides cushion and protection for internal organs
Necessary to provide essential fatty acids	Insulates our bodies against the cold
Enhances palatability by adding flavor and influencing texture of food	Reservoir of stored energy (100,000 calories in an average adult)
Provides satisfaction and a feeling of fullness	Necessary for hormone synthesis
Stimulates secretion of digestive juices	Essential component of all cells

Carbohydrate The Energy Nutrient

Does an active adult need more or fewer carbs? Most health experts support a plant-based diet high in carbohydrate (55%–60% of total calories), low in fat (15%–25% of total calories) and adequate in protein (20%–25% of total calories). Recently, however, these dietary recommendations have been challenged by individuals who argue that carbs need comprise only 40% or less of total calories with significantly larger amounts of calories coming from both fat and protein.

As a result, many fitness-minded people wonder if they should cut back on carbs. Not so fast! Decades of research have proven that diets rich in whole grains, vegetables and fruits help prevent disease, maintain weight and optimize athletic performance. Currently, no substantial evidence supports changing that recommendation.

Your body relies most on carbohydrates for fuel during exercise, and the amount you have stored affects your stamina and endurance. Carbs are stored as glycogen in limited amounts in muscles and the liver. Muscle glycogen is the fuel for your muscles, while liver glycogen maintains a normal blood-sugar level to fuel your brain. If your body depletes its glycogen stores, your blood sugar drops, and your brain struggles to control active muscles, causing you to experience mental fatigue and "hit the wall." Training and eating properly can increase your glycogen stores, and understanding the different types of carbs and how your body metabolizes them will help you reap the benefits of a high-carb diet.

When you eat a diet sufficient in carbs (50%–55% of calories or more), you have enough energy present in your muscles to fuel workouts and other activities completed within 90–120 minutes. On the other hand, during prolonged, strenuous exercise lasting more than two hours, taking in carbs at regular intervals is beneficial. For example, consuming 1 cup of a sports drink containing a 6%–10% carbohydrate concentration every 15–20 minutes can delay the onset of fatigue.

The best plan to improve your body is to work your muscles hard and fuel them optimally with a diet high in complex carbohydrates, adequate in protein and low in fat.

THE BODY RELIES MOST ON CARBOHYDRATES FOR FUEL DURING EXERCISE

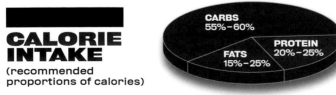

CALORIE INTAKE
(recommended proportions of calories)

CARBS 55%–60%

PROTEIN 20%–25%

FATS 15%–25%

Creative Carbs

>> If you're bored with white potatoes, try baking sweet potatoes or acorn squash.

>> For a filling lunch, slice boiled new potatoes over salads.

>> Raw sugar-snap peas make for a cool summer snack.

>> Explore the world of beans. Try combining one of the more than 20 different varieties with a grain-based food such as pasta or rice.

>> Try wild rice, brown rice, Spanish rice or long-grain rice.

>> Enjoy different whole-grain and multigrain breads spread with jam, honey or fruit butter.

Hydration Drink Up for Perfomance and Health

Long, tough workouts are not only exhaustive but can also be dangerous if you neglect to quench your thirst. Replacing the fluids you lose when you exercise is essential to sustaining performance, preventing dehydration and avoiding injury. What and when to drink is determined by how long and how hard you exercise and environmental conditions. For training and events less than one hour in duration, plain old water is sufficient for optimal rehydration. But workouts that last more than an hour increase fluid losses (1–2 quarts per hour) and drain your muscles' energy stores, making sports drinks the best way to replace fluids.

The three main ingredients of sports drinks — water, carbohydrate (6%–10%) and sodium — are precisely formulated for utilization during exercise. These drinks offset fluid loss, replace energy, boost fluid absorption into the blood and, of course, taste sweeter than water and have a range of flavors. If you dislike the taste, however, try diluting fruit juice, which is about 12%–15% carbohydrate, with an equal amount of water (1 cup juice with 1 cup water). The drawbacks of sports drinks are the cost and the excess calories, particularly if you're trying to lose weight. Taste-testing the different brands while you exercise will help you find a sports drink that works for you.

Keep in mind that these beverages aren't complete foods; they lack protein, fat, fiber and some essential vitamins and minerals. It's still necessary to eat a well-balanced diet that includes fruits, veggies, lean proteins, beans and grains to provide your body with the nutrients you need to perform your best.

More Fluid Facts and Guidelines

>> Drink before you're thirsty! Thirst isn't always a reliable indicator of fluid loss.

>> Drink fluids at a cool temperature. This helps regulate body temperature, cooling the inside of your body.

>> Unless you're an ultra-endurance athlete participating in events lasting more than eight hours, electrolyte (sodium, potassium and chloride) losses from exercise are easily overcome by typical intakes from the regular diet. Therefore, salt tablets and other electrolyte replacements aren't recommended.

HYPER-HYDRATE

>> Drink 2½ cups of water or a sports drink 1–2 hours before exercise.

>> Drink another 1½ cups of water or a sports drink for a total of 4 cups 15–30 minutes before exercise.

HYDRATE

>> Drink 1 cup of water or a sports drink every 15–20 minutes while you're exercising.

REHYDRATE

>> Weigh yourself before and after a workout. For each pound of weight lost, drink 2 cups of water. If you don't have a scale, drink until your urine is clear (a good indication of adequate hydration).

REPLACING THE FLUIDS LOST FROM YOUR BODY WHEN YOU EXERCISE IS ESSENTIAL TO SUSTAINING PERFORMANCE, PREVENTING DEHYDRATION AND AVOIDING INJURY

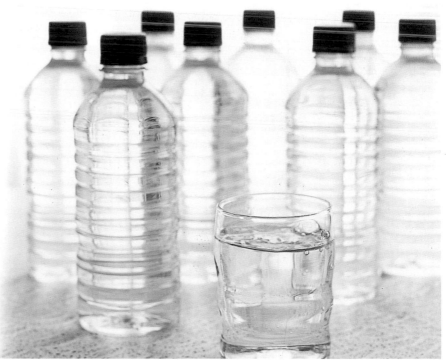

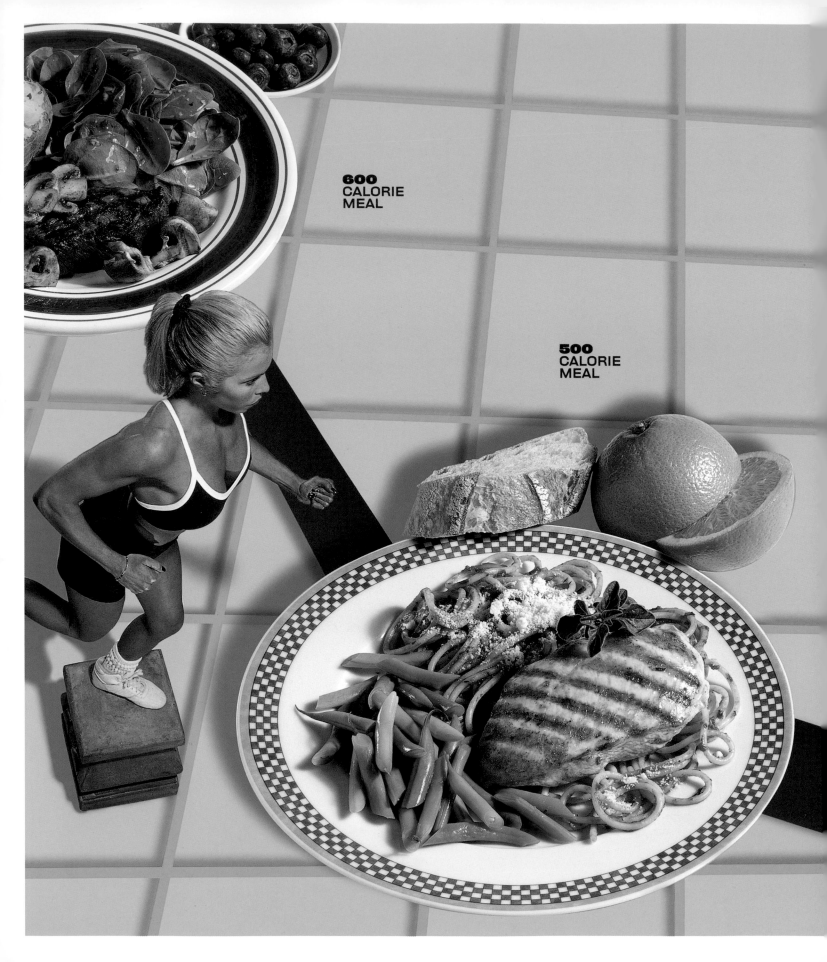

600
CALORIE
MEAL

500
CALORIE
MEAL

The Zigzag Diet

COUNTING THE CALORIC UPS AND DOWNS THAT CAN BOOST YOUR METABOLISM

Dieting is often the bane of the bodybuilder. How can you lose fat without losing muscle? With typical diets, you can't. You end up in a vicious cycle of repeated calorie cutting as your metabolism slows, making the shredded physique you crave seem unattainable. ¶ We have an approach that doesn't involve superstrict dieting or endless aerobic sessions. In fact, with this plan, on many days you eat a lot of food. Not only do you eat in a sensible manner, satisfying your palate and the mirror, but you can achieve permanent weight

control. You can do it with a technique called zigzag, or rotational, eating. This strategy involves judiciously increasing and decreasing your caloric consumption to stimulate your body's metabolism to burn fat while maintaining as much muscle as humanly possible. Best of all, it's easy to follow. Sound too good to be true? Keep reading to find out how to zigzag your way to a lean, muscular physique.

Tricking Your Metabolism

Typical dieting decreases not only bodyfat but also muscle mass. After a standard calorie-cutting program you'll weigh less (at least for a while), but you'll have a higher percentage of bodyfat than before because of the muscle you lost (your body will start to cannibalize amino acids from muscle for fuel). Even worse, once you return to a normal eating pattern, you're more likely to store additional calories as fat. The reason is that your body, in response to the decrease in calories, slows its metabolism to hold onto fat. The solution is to trick your body into believing it has a

surplus of food. In theory, this will keep your metabolism in a fat-burning, not fat-conserving, mode and at the same time hold onto the precious muscle you've been building.

While no specific research looks precisely at a zigzag approach to eating, we do have plenty of research that examines how the body responds to varying caloric intakes, macronutrient intakes and exercising. As an example, research from the Nutrition Research Centre at the University of Limburg, Maastricht, Netherlands, demonstrated that overfeeding increases sympathetic nervous system activity, accelerating the subjects' metabolism. Back in the States, researchers from the Pennington Biomedical Research Center and School of Human Ecology at Louisiana State University in Baton Rouge demonstrated that the human body adopts different energy utilization regimens dependent on eating a high-calorie or high-fat diet.

The fact that physiological changes also occur in response to high- and low-carbohydrate consumption won't cause you to fall over in amazement, nor will the news that different levels of

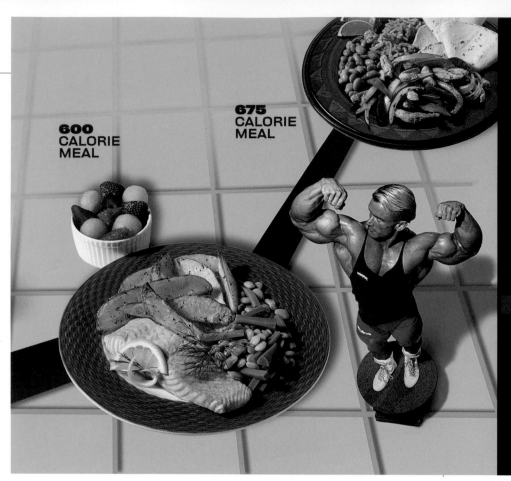

600 CALORIE MEAL

675 CALORIE MEAL

protein consumption elicit different responses. One study consisting of three days of fasting in six healthy young men found increased protein breakdown and oxidation of leucine during a very short time. Interestingly, this study also showed an 8% decrease in metabolic rate during the fasting period.

On the other end of the diet spectrum, overfeeding studies have shown that supercompensation with food results in increased lean body mass and blood levels of anabolic hormones. One study conducted in females demonstrated that a three-week period of overfeeding resulted in increased lean body mass and IGF-1, testosterone and insulin.

Eating Less Is Not Enough

The next step is to extrapolate from the research and try to find a way to make the physiological changes that occur in response to what and how much you eat work for you. But first let's discuss why just eating less may not be the best route. Simply cutting calories and protein, as in a standard diet, can cause reductions in growth hormone, IGF-1, insulin and androgens. This can certainly contribute to less than optimal muscle-building results.

With all this in mind, it would stand to reason that engaging in cycles of underfeeding and overfeeding, with brief periods of nutrient manipulation such as increasing and decreasing carbs, fats and protein, may result in an adaptive response that would

lead to less fat and more muscle. The benefits don't stop there. We all know that following a particular diet regimen can be boring, to put it mildly. Susan Kleiner, PhD, RD, nutritional consultant to many professional sports teams, faculty member at the University of Washington (Seattle) and author of *Power Eating* (Human Kinetics, 1998) views a rotational diet strategy as beneficial. "Many bodybuilders engage in severe dieting strategies," she says. "At times they may find it difficult to make it through the week. Having the ability to switch gears and change your eating habits for a little while can provide, if nothing else, a tremendous psychological boost."

The Program

Clearly, the key to staying lean isn't excessive dieting but rather developing an eating strategy that's easy to follow and fits your lifestyle. Get off the losing-and-gaining-it-all-back roller coaster. Set your sights on balance and sensibility regarding food and getting lean. Zigzag, or rotational, eating allows you to manipulate calories on a weekly basis to make yourself a muscle-building, fat-burning machine — for life.

>> **Calorie Counting:** To begin the program, you need to determine how many calories you consume on an average day. Keep a seven-day food record by writing down everything you eat in one week, then add up the total calories and divide by seven

"CUT YOUR CALORIES GRADUALLY, THEN BEFORE YOUR METABOLISM ADJUSTS TO THE LOWER-CALORIE INTAKE...ZIGZAG YOUR CALORIES UP BEFORE YOU CUT BACK AGAIN"

to get your daily average. For example, if you consumed 17,500 calories in a week, that averages out to 2,500 per day. That's how many calories you need to maintain your current weight. We'll use this as a starting point for the zigzag.

>> How to Eat: After calculating your daily calorie intake, the next step is to determine the amount of fat, protein and carbs you eat each day. Fat is especially important to keep track of because it contributes 9 calories per gram, more than both carbohydrate and protein (4 calories per gram each). To get lean, a great place to begin cutting calories is with your fat intake. As a general guideline for bodybuilders, keep your fat consumption around 15% of your daily calories.

Of course, protein is absolutely vital when trying to maintain lean body mass while dropping bodyfat. Quality sources of protein include skinless chicken breast, fish, turkey breast, egg whites, lean beef and whey protein powder. Your protein intake should be about 1 gram per pound of bodyweight each day.

While protein is essential to the growth and preservation of muscle, carbohydrates provide the fuel you need to pump iron. If your body doesn't have carbohydrate available for energy, it won't hesitate to tap into muscle tissue for energy substrates. Carbs should come from foods like oatmeal, whole-grain bread, rice, pasta, potatoes and fruit. Avoid highly processed carb sources like sweetened drinks and baked goods. About 3 grams of carbs for each pound of bodyweight daily should do, adjusted up or down depending on whether you're in a higher- or lower-calorie phase.

>> Slash and Burn: To lose bodyfat you'll need to create a caloric deficit, but you'll be cutting calories with a twist. The zigzag works by manipulating your body's natural tendency to slow its metabolic rate in response to perceived starvation. By systematically decreasing and then increasing calories, you can exploit this survival mechanism to your advantage: preventing plateaus in fat loss while preserving skeletal muscle.

Preserving muscle is key because that's the metabolic regulator for your body. The more lean body mass you have, the more calories you burn at rest and during exercise. Keep in mind that muscle is living tissue and burns calories like an inferno. If you want low bodyfat, you must keep as much muscle as possible.

Putting the Zigzag to Work

With your average caloric intake in hand, begin a gradual cutback in calories. The drop is slow, taking six weeks to achieve the goal of a 500-calorie-per-day reduction. To maintain a maximum amount of muscle, focus on slow and steady progress. Plan to eat 4–6 meals per day, depending on your schedule. These frequent meals let you split up your calories more evenly during the day and keep energy levels high, while providing a steady influx of amino acids for hard-working muscles.

Begin with a 300-calorie decrease by cutting down on high-fat condiments like salad dressings, mayonnaise, butter and margarine. After four weeks, cut an additional 200 calories per day, making the total decrease 500 calories.

After two weeks with the 500-calorie deficit, begin the zigzag. As your metabolism begins to slow, simply increase your calories by about 200 calories for about three days, then drop them back down to the deficit level for a week. This is only a general recommendation; since the timing is so important, you need to make sure that you hit it just right for you. Try some slightly different time frames to see how you respond.

The additional calories should come in the form of complex carbs. Spread them over your first three meals of the day, making sure one of those high-carb meals comes after you train. Consider scheduling your high-carb days when training big muscle groups like legs and back. This keeps the body from getting overtrained due to chronic caloric restriction.

Permanent Fix

To make the zigzag work, you need to take the time required. If you want to stay lean and muscular year round, you have to permanently alter your metabolic rate and body composition. And the only way to do that is by maintaining muscle while cutting fat. You may even add skeletal muscle during periods of fat loss while zigzag dieting.

The zigzag program isn't a diet to get on, then fall off a few months later. It's a new approach to getting lean, one scientifically based on cycling your food intake to tap into your body's hidden potential to burn fat. *(See references on page 164)*

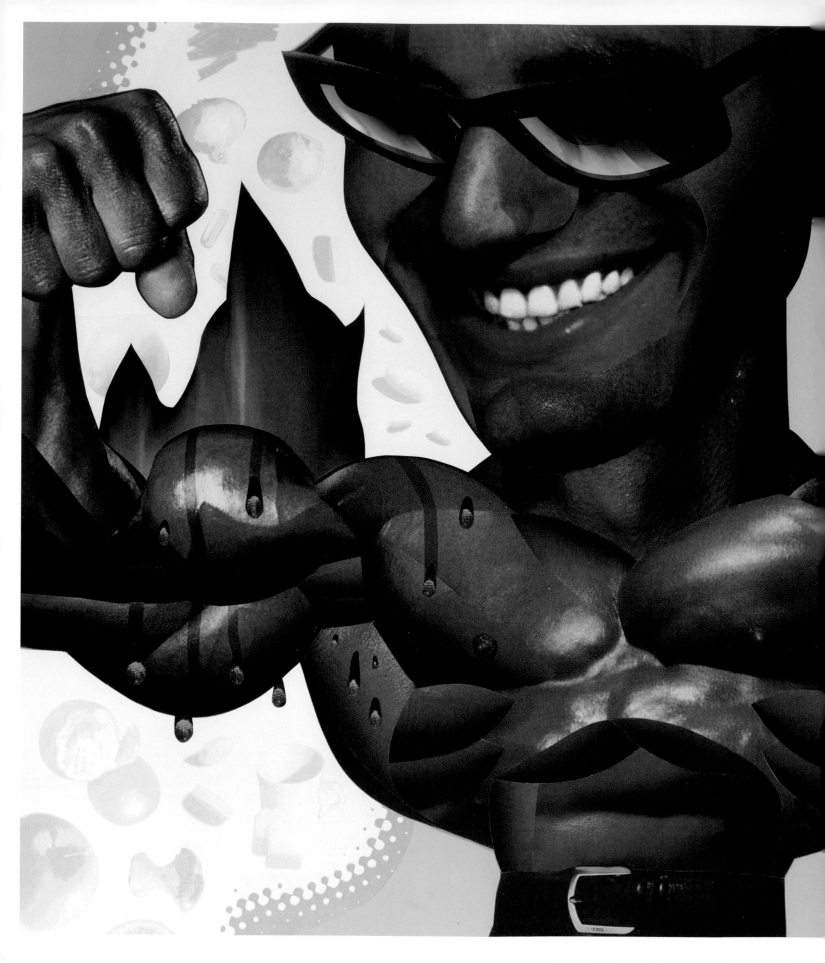

Fat-Loss Power Pills

THESE EPHEDRINE-FREE SUPPLEMENTS CAN HELP YOU GET LEAN FASTER

Picture this: It's summer and you're at the beach, looking for the perfect spot. Up ahead, you see an opening in the sea of half-naked bodies and hustle over to stake your claim. As you approach you realize your luck — to the left, three gorgeous females who could give the cast of "Charlie's Angels" a run for their money; to the right, two more hotties in bikinis that would be illegal in some states. You set up camp and the women periodically check you out as you nonchalantly pull off your T-shirt to reveal your chiseled body. The fruits of

your labor have definitely paid off, big time....

Now, unfortunately, we must return to the present. Your fat, out-of-shape present. To fast-forward to the lean, muscular body that'll have all the girls at the beach paying attention to you this summer, you have to step into diet mode, pump up your lifting intensity and crank out the cardio. You should also consider one more detail: fat-burning supplements.

The added boost from supplements can make all the difference at the end of the day. Although ephedrine was an effective tool, it's now an extinct ingredient. Luckily, many new kids on the supplement block can deliver the same, if not better, results, if you know how to combine them for faster fat-burning power.

Most fat-burning supplements can be separated into two categories, based on their primary method of attacking fat. The first group is the central nervous system (CNS) supplements, which work via the neurotransmitters produced by the CNS. They either increase the production of those neurotransmitters, enhance their actions or mimic them altogether. The second

group consists of the thyroid-stimulating fat-burners. These supplements work to enhance the production and/or action of the thyroid hormones, most importantly T3.

[CNS FAT-FIGHTERS]

Synephrine

To fill the big shoes left vacant by ephedrine, supplement scientists employed a compound with a similar structure and action known as synephrine — an extract from the bitter orange fruit (*Citrus aurantium*) that may be listed on product labels as *Zhi shi*.

Synephrine mimics the actions of the natural neurotransmitter norepinephrine (similar to adrenaline), which works to increase metabolic rate and heart rate. Studies show that synephrine significantly increases metabolic rate and fat loss similar to, although somewhat weaker than, ephedrine. But also weaker is synephrine's effect on the cardiovascular system, as it barely raises blood pressure and heart rate.

>> How to Optimize: Look for products that deliver a dose of 5–20 mg of synephrine (from a standardized *Citrus aurantium* extract) and take once or twice per day for a maximum of 40 mg per day.

>> Keep in Mind: As with ephedrine and other fat-burners, the effect from synephrine is enhanced when caffeine is also used. But because it does have a mild effect on the cardiovascular system, don't take it if you have a history of cardiovascular problems or if you're taking antidepressants or other MAO inhibitors.

Octopamine

Similar to synephrine, octopamine is another extract from *Citrus aurantium*. Octopamine has been shown in the lab to specifically target receptors found on fat cells that cause fat cells to shrink. Research on the effects of octopamine on fat loss is sparse, but some anecdotal evidence supports its effectiveness at high doses. A definite benefit of octopamine is the fact that it appears to lack any effect on heart rate or blood pressure.

>> How to Optimize: Because octopamine's effectiveness is dose-dependent, you'll need to use products that provide at least 150–250 mg of octopamine per dose. Take it 1–3 times per day.

>> Keep in Mind: Although octopamine itself doesn't appear to affect the cardiovascular system, most products with octopamine also contain some synephrine. This means that individuals with a history of cardiovascular problems or who take MAO inhibitors should avoid products containing octopamine.

Tyrosine

The amino acid tyrosine is used by the body to make a number of important hormones and neurotransmitters, including norepinephrine (NE), dopamine and the thyroid hormones (T3 and T4). Research studies in humans confirm that dietary tyrosine increases NE levels, which makes it a perfect supplement to take with NE mimickers like synephrine. The enhanced NE levels also provide a direct effect on the brain to control appetite.

>> How to Optimize: Most fat-burners that throw tyrosine in the mix can't jam enough into the tablets or capsules to make a huge difference. If your brand doesn't list the amount of tyrosine on the label, assume it's less than 500 mg. You'll need a minimum of 500 mg, but will get much more from about 1,000–2,000 mg taken as two divided doses. We recommend buying tyrosine capsules and popping them with your fat-burner to make up the difference.

>> Keep in Mind: Bumping up your levels of NE can give some people the jitters and cause nausea in others unless a "slow and steady" dosing schedule is used. Start off at around 500 mg and increase as your tolerance allows. Don't take tyrosine if you have skin cancer, as it may speed the growth of this type of tumor. You should also avoid it if you have a mood or bipolar disorder.

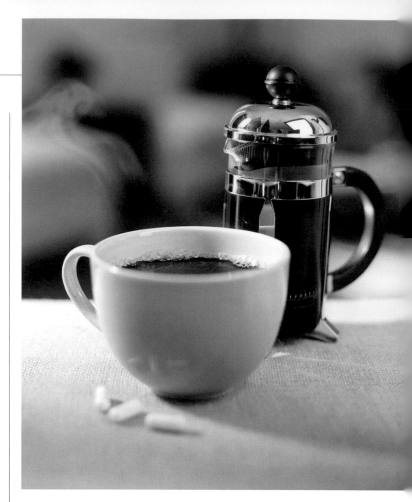

Green Tea Extract

Green tea contains several compounds called catechins; the main one responsible for its thermogenic and antioxidant properties is epigallocatechin gallate (EGCG). Green tea's fat-burning ability is well supported by scientific studies that suggest an increase in metabolic rate of more than 4%. For many guys, this will amount to almost 150 extra calories burned per day. (It may not seem like much, but every little bit helps.) The key is combining several ingredients — as most fat-burning products do — to up the fat-burning ante, in addition to smart eating and exercise for the fastest fat loss. Although scientists originally theorized that the caffeine in green tea caused the fat-burning effect, they now realize EGCG may inhibit the enzyme responsible for the degradation of NE. This allows NE's fat-burning effect to be stronger and last longer, making EGCG a perfect add-on ingredient to go with tyrosine and NE-mimicking supplements.

>> How to Optimize: You'll need to get about 90 mg of EGCG or 270 mg of polyphenols per dose. Take this amount 2–3 times per day.

>> Keep in Mind: EGCG delays blood clotting, so it's best to avoid taking green tea extract before surgery or while taking blood-thinning or anti-inflammatory drugs (this interaction is even more likely if you're also taking Vitamin E, fish oil or ginkgo biloba as part of your supplement regimen).

THE KEY IS COMBINING SEVERAL INGREDIENTS TO UP THE FAT-BURNING ANTE, IN ADDITION TO SMART EATING AND EXERCISE FOR THE FASTEST FAT LOSS

Caffeine

Although it's a natural ingredient, caffeine is considered the most popular drug in the world. This "wake-me-up" molecule found in coffee, tea, sodas, chocolate, and herbs like guarana and mate does more than boost your energy — it enhances the use of fat as fuel by increasing epinephrine (adrenaline) and NE release, particularly during exercise, and enhances the effectiveness of other fat-burning ingredients. Caffeine in moderate doses is now believed to lower the risk for developing type II diabetes, obesity, cancer and heart disease. Recent studies suggest that pure caffeine is more effective for fat loss than the natural form in coffee.

>> **How to Optimize:** Get about 100–300 mg of caffeine per dose. Take 1–2 times per day. To optimize fat loss, take one dose within a two-hour window of your workout.

Yohimbine

Yohimbine is the active ingredient found in the African tree *Pausinystalia yohimbe*. Although commonly used to enhance male libido, it enhances fat-burning by inhibiting the alpha-adrenoreceptors found on fat cells (adipocytes) that work to limit the amount of fat leaving those cells. By antagonizing the alpha-adrenoreceptors, yohimbe allows the adipocytes to more easily release their stores of fatty acids for energy and makes it more difficult for them to store fat. The fat-mobilizing effect of yohimbine is enhanced if taken in combination with caffeine.

>> **How to Optimize:** Take supplements containing standardized yohimbe extract that provide about 5–10 mg of yohimbine once in the morning and once at night.

>> **Keep in Mind:** Don't take yohimbe products if you take MAO inhibitors or have a history of high blood pressure, diabetes, glaucoma or mental disturbance, especially bipolar disorder.

[THYROID THERMOGENICS]

Forskolin

Coleus forskohlii is an herb containing the active ingredient forskolin, which has been shown in scientific studies to increase thyroid hormone production. The thyroid hormones, particularly T3, play a major role in regulating the metabolic rate of the cells. Forskolin also activates fat breakdown from within the fat cell and has a muscle-preserving effect, which can be critical when dieting. Unlike some of the CNS supplements, forskolin actually causes an overall drop in blood pressure, which could be good for those with elevated blood pressure and those who want to counter the effects of caffeine and synephrine.

>> **How to Optimize:** Take *Coleus forskohlii* supplements that deliver 20–50 mg of actual forskolin 2–3 times per day.

>> **Keep in Mind:** Avoid getting more than 150 mg of total forskolin per day, and don't take it if you have a heart condition, thyroid disorder or prostate cancer.

Guggulsterones

Guggulsterones are plant sterols extracted from the resin of the *Commiphora mukul* tree grown in India. While there are many guggulsterone compounds in this resin, it's the E and Z guggulsterones that have the highest degree of human bioactivity and have been shown in studies to affect thyroid hormone production, cholesterol levels and even acne.

>> **How to Optimize:** Look for products that deliver about 20–60 mg of guggulsterones E and Z and take 1–3 times per day.

>> **Keep in Mind:** Always be sure to consult your physician before taking any guggulsterone product if you have a thyroid disorder.

7-Keto

3-acetyl-7-Oxo DHEA (7-keto DHEA) is a natural metabolite of dehydroepiandrosterone (DHEA), the hormone produced by the adrenal glands to form testosterone. But unlike DHEA, 7-keto DHEA doesn't convert to testosterone or estrogens. It increases metabolic rate through an increase in thyroid hormone production. As an added fat-burning bonus, it also appears to directly enhance metabolism at the mitochondria (aerobic energy factories within cells).

>> **How to Optimize:** Try 100–200 mg of 7-keto DHEA per day, taken as 1–3 divided doses.

>> **Keep in Mind:** Consult a physician before taking 7-keto if you have a thyroid disorder.

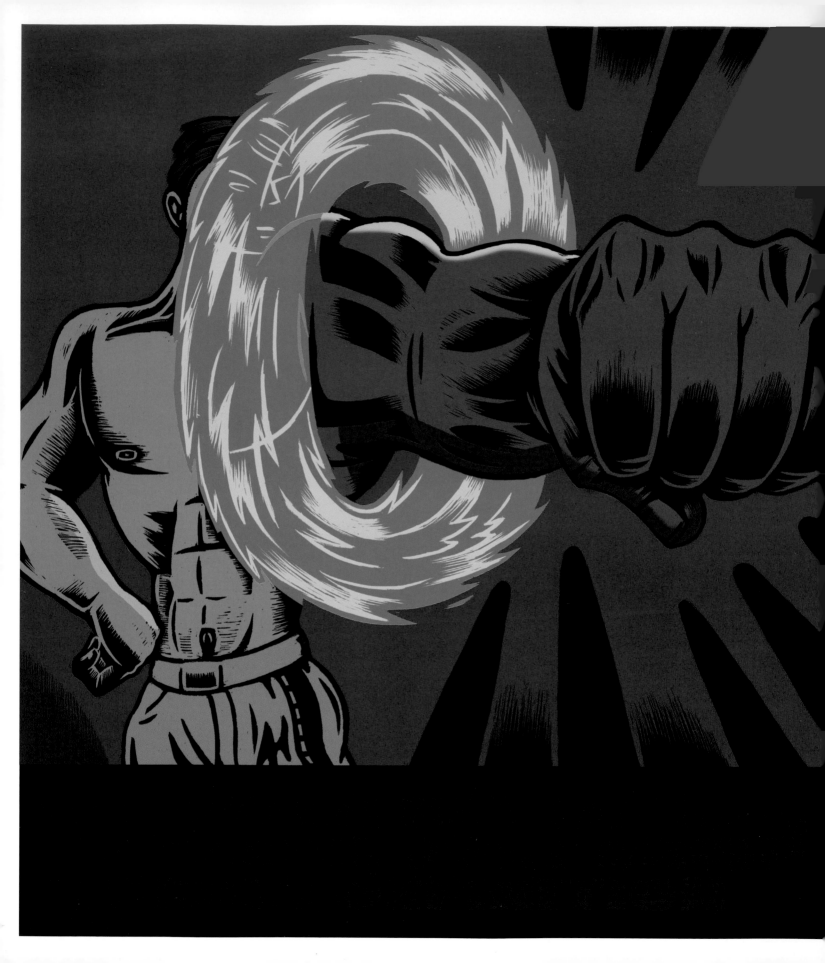

One Week to Peak

OVERHAUL YOUR PHYSIQUE IN EIGHT DAYS WITH THIS DIET AND TRAINING PLAN

Is it possible to radically transform your physique in just over a week? Can you really overhaul your appearance in eight days, going from soft to downright ripped? Yep, provided you're already in decent shape. In fact, competitive bodybuilders do it every time they compete. ¶ You can, too, with this "how-to" guide to manipulating four factors: carbohydrates, exercise, sodium and water. When tweaked precisely, the result is a temporary super-hard look on par with that of a dialed-in bodybuilder. No water retention, no bloating, just crisp definition. Competitive bodybuilders are notorious for radically changing their physiques in as few as 7–9 days. During the final stretch before

a competition, many follow a system called "carbohydrate depleting and loading." This involves radically restricting your carbs, then reverting back to a very high carb intake. The process empties the muscles of their carbohydrate reserves only to load them back up. (Other players in the transformation process include altering training styles and manipulating your sodium and water intake.)

You'll need to eat clean throughout the week: no fast food or processed foods and limited dietary fat (see "Day in the Life" on page 141 for sample meal plans). Increase your protein intake as well, to 1½–2 grams per pound of bodyweight a day.

Here, we give you a Friday-to-Friday plan for a complete physique overhaul and rapid transformation. Use it as a quick fix before a trip to the beach or a weekend cruise. We just hope you recognize yourself in the mirror when you're done.

1) Start Phase Friday–Tuesday

>> Salt Your Food

Salt makes you retain water, right? True, but manipulating its intake can lead to water loss. Here's how: Two days before depleting carbs, add table salt or spices made with salt to each of your meals — enough to make the food taste salty — because salt causes temporary water retention. When you eliminate salt completely but keep drinking water, the result is extreme water excretion.

>> Up Your Water

As you increase salt, you'll want to increase your water intake (distilled water, if possible); 5–7 glasses more than your normal daily intake will suffice. The added water preps your body. Then, when you restrict water the final two days, the change in intake creates the illusion of a water deficit. Low water levels, especially under your skin, make you look more ripped.

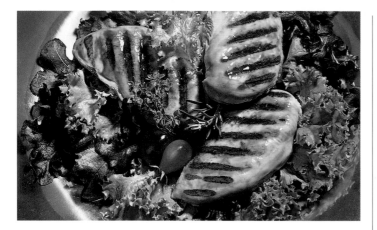

2) Depleting Phase Sunday–Tuesday

>> Cut Your Carbs

This step brings the entire system together. Reduce your carbohydrates to 40–70 grams a day for three consecutive days to burn the stored glycogen out of your muscles. Simultaneously, train with higher reps (12–15 per set) and increase the number of sets you perform by 50%. For example, if you do 12 sets for chest, up that to 18 sets. This combination fully depletes your muscles of glycogen.

3) Loading Phase Wednesday–Friday

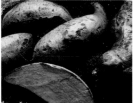

>> Load Up on Carbs

In the reverse of Step 2, increase your carb intake to 2½–3½ grams per pound of bodyweight daily. (A 200-pound male would need at least 500–700 grams a day.) Since training depletes carbs, you'll skip it altogether, allowing all incoming carbohydrates to be stockpiled as muscle glycogen. When glycogen stores are excessively low and a high-carb intake is reintroduced, muscles store more glycogen than ever before.

>> Drop the Salt

When you stop salting your food, water will be readily lost, promoting better definition. Eliminate all refined foods.

>> Drop Your Water

When your muscles begin filling back up with glycogen, water is required. When you cut back to half your *normal* intake, a lot of the water required to make glycogen is dragged from beneath your skin and stored in your muscles, creating less water retention and clear definition.

>> Scratch the Training

Training while carb-loading will siphon off the carbs stored in your muscles, which you don't want. Don't train on these days. Sit back and watch in awe as your body tightens.

(*See reference on page 164*)

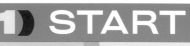

1) START

Here is your at-a-glance Friday-to-Friday guide to peaking, outlining how you'll manipulate salt, water, carbs and training on a daily basis.

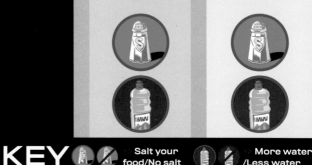

KEY — Salt your food/No salt · More water/Less water

GLUTAMINE & POTASSIUM: THE RIGHT SUPPLEMENTS FOR YOUR PEAKING WEEK

Depleting carbs sets up a reaction in which your body begins to make all kinds of enzymes to create new muscle glycogen. When you load — and the glycogen-forming machinery is stoked — you can store more muscle glycogen than ever. Two nutrients that can help are glutamine and potassium.

>> Taking 5 grams of glutamine three times a day during a loading phase (days 6, 7 and 8) can result in better glycogen storage. Try mixing it into a carbohydrate drink.

>> Potassium helps make glycogen and draws water inside your muscle cells. The more water within your cells, the less likely it is to be stored beneath your skin. Try taking 1,000 mg of supplemental potassium daily (200 mg with each of any five meals) during the entire eight days.

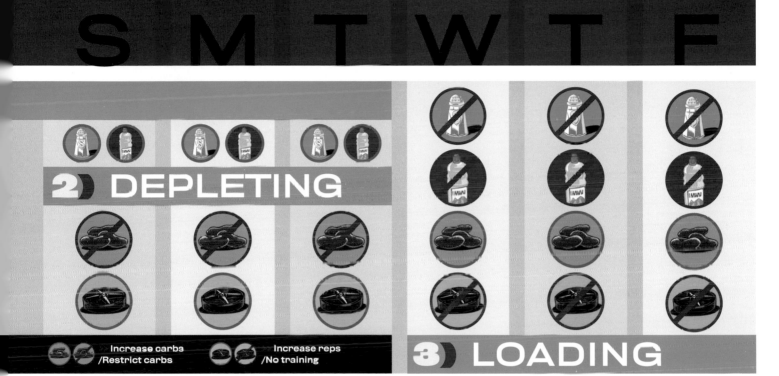

DAY IN THE LIFE

DEPLETING – A SAMPLE DAY OF EATING FROM SUNDAY THROUGH TUESDAY FOR THE 200-POUNDER

LOADING – A SAMPLE DAY OF EATING FROM WEDNESDAY THROUGH FRIDAY NO. 2 FOR THE 200-POUNDER

MEAL 1
8 egg whites,
 2 yolks
Salt and pepper
1 cup mushrooms
3 glasses water

MEAL 2
10 oz. chicken
 breast
Mixed green salad
 with no-carb dressing
3 glasses water

MEAL 3
8 oz. lean steak
 with Cajun
 spices
2 cups green beans
3 glasses water

MEAL 4
Whey protein
 drink made
 with 2 glasses
 water

MEAL 5
1 rounded cup
 low-fat cottage
 cheese
2 glasses water

MEAL 6
10 oz. chicken
 breast with salt
 or lemon-pepper
 seasoning that
 contains salt
1 cup broccoli
2 glasses water

MEAL 1
6 oz. lean steak
2 12-oz. potatoes,
 shredded and
 grilled with
 nonstick
 cooking spray
1 glass water

MEAL 2
10 oz. chicken
 breast
12 oz. yam
1 glass water

MEAL 3
8 oz. lean steak
2 yams
1 cup green beans
No water

MEAL 4
10 oz. chicken breast
2 12-oz. potatoes
1 glass water

MEAL 5
8 oz. turkey
 breast
2 yams
No water

MEAL 6
10 oz. chicken
 breast
2 12-oz. potatoes
1 cup broccoli
1 glass water

MEAL 7
1 yam

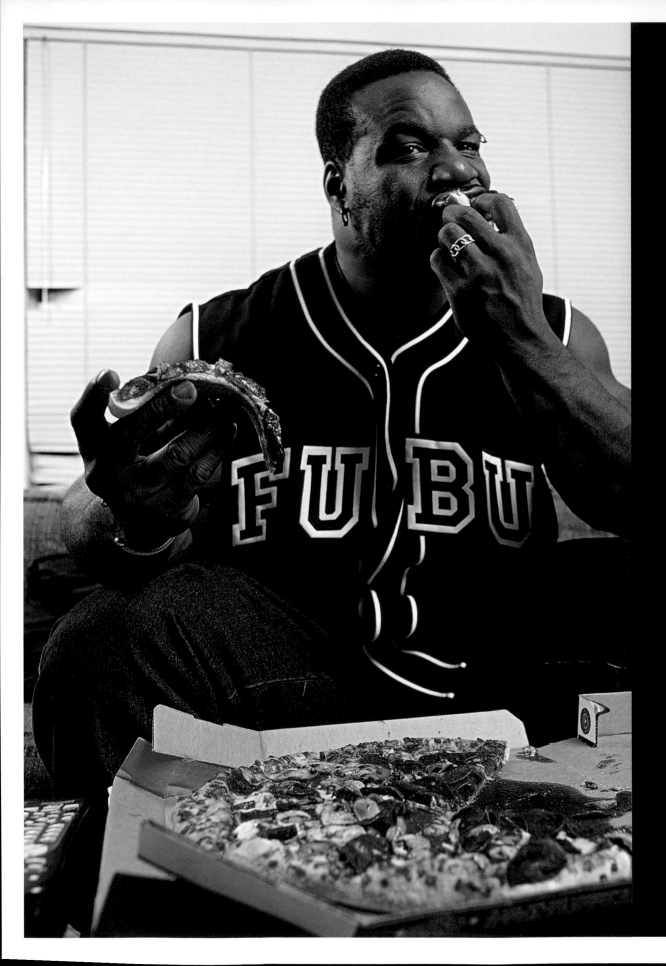

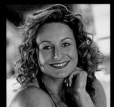

LOVENA STAMATIOU-TULEY
Lawrence, Kansas. Physical therapist and IFBB pro fitness competitor

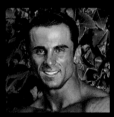

WILL DUGGAN
Los Angeles. Electrical engineer and NPC bodybuilder

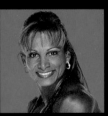

ADELA GARCIA-FRIEDMANSKY
Normal, Illinois. Personal trainer, Spinning and aerobics instructor and IFBB pro fitness competitor

Thinkin' Lean

GET YOUR HEAD IN THE GAME IF YOU WANT TO SEE SUCCESS ON THE SCALE

What do you do when your meal plan says tuna but your stomach says cake? Three superfit dieters show you the mental strategies you should adopt if you want to stick to a healthy nutrition program.

M&F: What's the first thing you do to mentally prepare for a diet?

WILL: It definitely has to be gradual. You can't jump in with both feet and just pick up on a strict diet or you'll go into shell-shock. Slowly you want to cut out the sweets and fats and other carbohydrates, probably in that order. For example, I like to have a few slices of fat-free cheese on my egg whites when I'm getting into diet mode. But I'll transition to having the egg whites alone. This way your body doesn't starve and it doesn't freak out on you. It's kind of difficult the first week or two, but after that you just get into a rhythm.

M&F: Is dieting more inspiration or perspiration?

WILL: In all honesty, you can't have one without the other and be successful. Both are probably equally important; I'd put them both at 50% since they're contingent on each other.

Getting results is so much about diet. A lot of people think it's just training. They think they can go beat the heck out of themselves in the gym and see results when their diet is terrible. Many people just aren't diligent in their diet; they don't put in the time or dedication to cook and prepare the food, bring a lunchbox and so on.

I carry a huge cooler everywhere and get teased all the time. Everyone else brings a tiny cooler, but mine could hold a case of beer and a couple of steaks. I prepare my food at home and put it in Tupperware so all I have to do is heat it in the microwave.

My boss comes around and asks: "You're eating again? If you'd work as much as you eat, we'd all be rich around here." But it's all good-natured because he sees some of the successes I'm having.

LOVENA: My answer is both. Like any goal-setting or business plan, just getting started is the hardest part. However, as you start to achieve your short-term goals and you see progress being made, you feel empowered. This inspires you to continue, and the process becomes easier both mentally and physically.

It's the same with dieting and working out. Visualize, set goals, have a plan, and stay the course with determination and confidence. Of course, a whole lot of positive self-talk and a supportive environment help, too!

Mind Games

M&F: Do you rely on any mental rituals to help you get through the day?

ADELA: While I'm doing my cardio in the morning, I try to concentrate on what I have to do to stay focused. That's especially important when I start getting closer to a show because it gets a little harder when your energy level is so low. The main thing is keeping your mind in the game.

WILL: I wake up at about 4:15 or 4:30 and stumble downstairs for an hour of cardio on my stationary bike. The bike's in the living room, where I have about 10 years of trophies and some magazine covers I've had. Just being in the room motivates me. I'll imagine who's going to be next to me onstage and think, *I'm sure they're in bed right now.* So that makes me feel good because I don't know a lot of people who will wake up at 4:15.

M&F: Is it hard being at work when no one else is dieting like you are? Do your co-workers bring in junk food all the time?

LOVENA: That's what I deal with. I'm very much alone and have been alone since starting my career, as far as being in Kansas and trying to be serious about fitness. People might say, "Oh, you're so extreme," or "One bite won't kill you."

I take a blender to work and everybody can hear it, so that's a problem. So then I try to make egg whites and everybody can smell them. Even people in my gym aren't as into fitness as people are probably anywhere along the coasts of the U.S.

The wonderful thing is, I've started coaching girls for fitness in the last couple of years. I finally have at least some women around me who have similar goals. Somebody to hold me accountable and who doesn't think it's so bizarre that I eat the way I do.

WILL: There's always someone bringing in doughnuts every morning. There aren't a lot of people here who work out. So they kind of look at me like a science project gone awry, but in the same sense, it separates me and makes me feel good. You need mental strength as well as physical strength, and I like to have this balance in life.

Temptation Alley

M&F: How do you deal with tempting foods like the daily dozen doughnuts?

WILL: I keep posters of the show that I'm doing in my office. I'll tell myself that the people who'll be onstage with me aren't going to eat that right now, so if I eat it, I'll be behind them.

M&F: When you're craving a tempting food, is it better for you to have just one bite or avoid it completely?

WILL: I definitely wouldn't even touch it. Once you cross that line, your mouth starts watering and you start thinking about it. It's just better for me not to do it at all, and that's probably what I'd recommend to anybody else. One bite's not going to satisfy you anyway, it's just going to make you want more.

ADELA: Once you give in to one bite, you're going to want more. It's not like you're really going to have just one cookie, or one bite of cheesecake or ice cream. If I want to have something bad, normally I just look at myself in the mirror and ask, *Do I really want to ruin what I've done so far?* Because it takes so much work to get where you're at.

LOVENA: The moment you have a bite or a taste, it's like opening up Pandora's Box. That's mentally hard. I know a lot of girls who are better at moderation and can have a little bit of

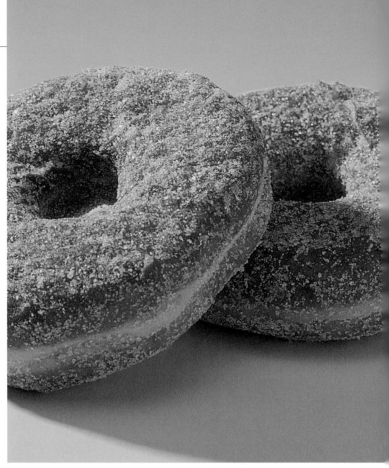

something, but I'm just not. I'm either on or off. I don't want to play with fire; I don't believe in "kind of" dieting. It just doesn't work for me.

Cheaters Can Prosper

M&F: Do you have a cheat day?

ADELA: My trainer wants me to have a cheat day. I've noticed that cheating actually helps me a little bit. Before one show, my trainer told me I could have steak and a baked potato on my cheat day. I thought to myself, *But that's just eating normally.* Instead I had pizza and ice cream and I actually lost a couple of pounds.

WILL: I do cheat on Sundays when I'm getting ready for a show. A lot of people I know cheat the whole day, but I usually just cheat for one meal. I won't junk out on pizza and burgers; instead I'll go out for some sushi. It's the carbs that my body craves; I'm not real big on candy and sweets. Even then, before I go I'll usually have a protein shake just so I don't overdo it.

Keep It Clean

M&F: Is it easier to eat clean year-round or take a break in the off-season?

ADELA: Normally I'm not so strict during the off-season, but I still try to eat fairly clean. I'll have bread, cottage cheese, a lot of fruit, and I'm allowed at least three cheat meals per week.

"ONE BITE'S NOT GOING TO SATISFY YOU ANYWAY, IT'S JUST GOING TO MAKE YOU WANT MORE. — WILL"

I actually like eating clean. I have a blood condition that requires me to eat healthy — my white blood cells are low, a condition that runs in my family. I don't feel very good if I eat something without a lot of high-density nutrients.

People ask me if I ever get tired of eating [clean] and I say no, sometimes I miss it. When I take a week or so off after a show and eat whatever I want, my body just doesn't feel right. You enjoy it for a week but then you don't feel very good afterward.

WILL: During the off-season I eat probably three or four clean meals a day, then I'll go ahead and enjoy a piece of pizza or hamburger once in a while. But I train hard enough and intense enough, with focus and discipline, that I don't really get fat. I know you have to put on some size and with that comes the fat and water, but you still want to look halfway decent. The bigger you blow up, the harder it is to come down again.

LOVENA: I'll eat out more and still try to make healthy choices, so you won't usually see me ordering stuff straight off the menu. I usually try to modify it a little.

If I decide to mess up, I'm going to mess up all the way. I'll eat really well and then have the cheesecake. I'm going to pick and choose and let myself have this fabulous dessert that I can really enjoy and appreciate.

M&F: What's the biggest challenge of sticking to a diet?

WILL: When I first started, eating clean every single day was just a whole other world. I'd basically survived my whole life on junk food and sweets at least a couple of times a week, if not every day. In the beginning I could have named 20 foods I missed. Now the hardest thing is probably the transition between the off-season and diet mode. That week or so, you basically say, *Okay, now it's time to get down to business.* Now it doesn't take me as long to acclimate because I've been doing it quite a while, but I still feel it. After you start seeing results, though, your motivation kind of snowballs.

Secret of Success

M&F: Is it incredible willpower that lets you stick with your program, or something more?

WILL: If you train your mind, there isn't anything in this world that you can't accomplish. You have to learn to break out of that comfort zone and to operate in turbulent waters. Willpower is definitely a key element, but overall, it's your entire mind-set and determination to succeed that will make you prevail.

M&F: What do you say to yourself when the going gets tough and you're tempted to give in . . . sleep in . . . or dig in?

ADELA: I tell myself to keep my mind on the goal. I think about what the other girls are doing: If I'm working hard, somebody else is working harder. You have to stay on track with your training and nutrition and don't let anything take you away from that. If you do, it's going to show when you step onstage — you don't want them looking at your booty.

LOVENA: When I'm hitting that snooze button for the third time, it always comes back down to, you know, *How bad do you want it?* If I'm preparing for a competition, I'll add, *So and so's probably getting out of bed, so get your butt out of bed.*

Words of Wisdom

M&F: We've talked a lot about competition. What would you say to people who want to get in great shape but aren't competing in a bodybuilding or fitness show?

LOVENA: When I'm not competing, the truth is that I feel the same way. Half the time you're at the gym thinking, *Oh, I really don't like the way that looks.* So I think, *You know, if you don't like it, then do something about it. You had your fun and now it's time to pay the piper.*

WILL: I'd advise them to put an inspirational figure up on their wall, refrigerator, whatever. Someone or something that motivates them so they won't deviate on a tangent.

As far as breaking the diet goes, you just have to either do it 100% or not do it at all. That's kind of my philosophy on life. I know it may be a bit extreme for some, but when someone procrastinates and makes excuses, it's that much easier to keep doing it the next time and the time after that.

I'm actually an engineer before I'm a bodybuilder; I don't have any ambitions of turning pro. Bodybuilding is a complement to my life and a way to have some goals. It's something you can carry with you day in and day out and always feel good about.

[CHAPTER SIX]

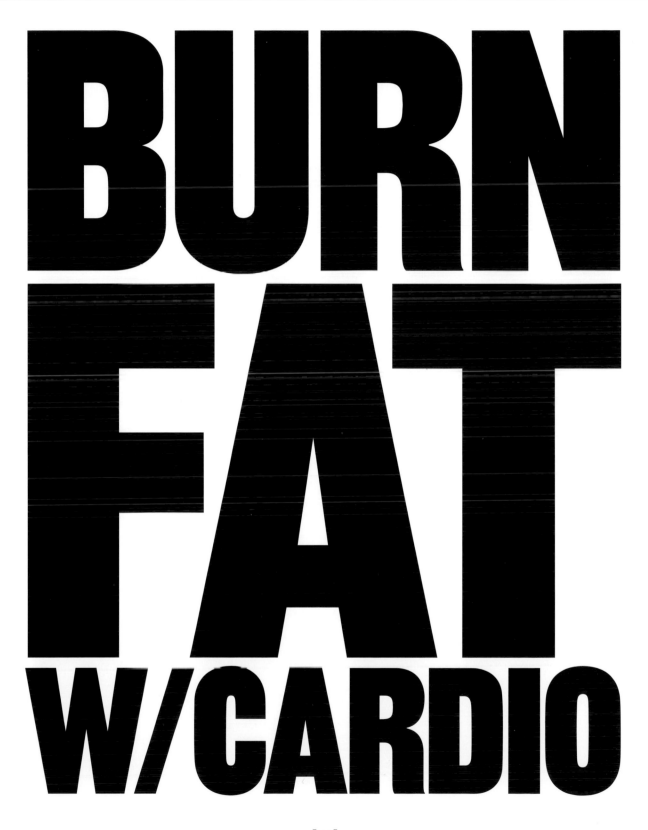

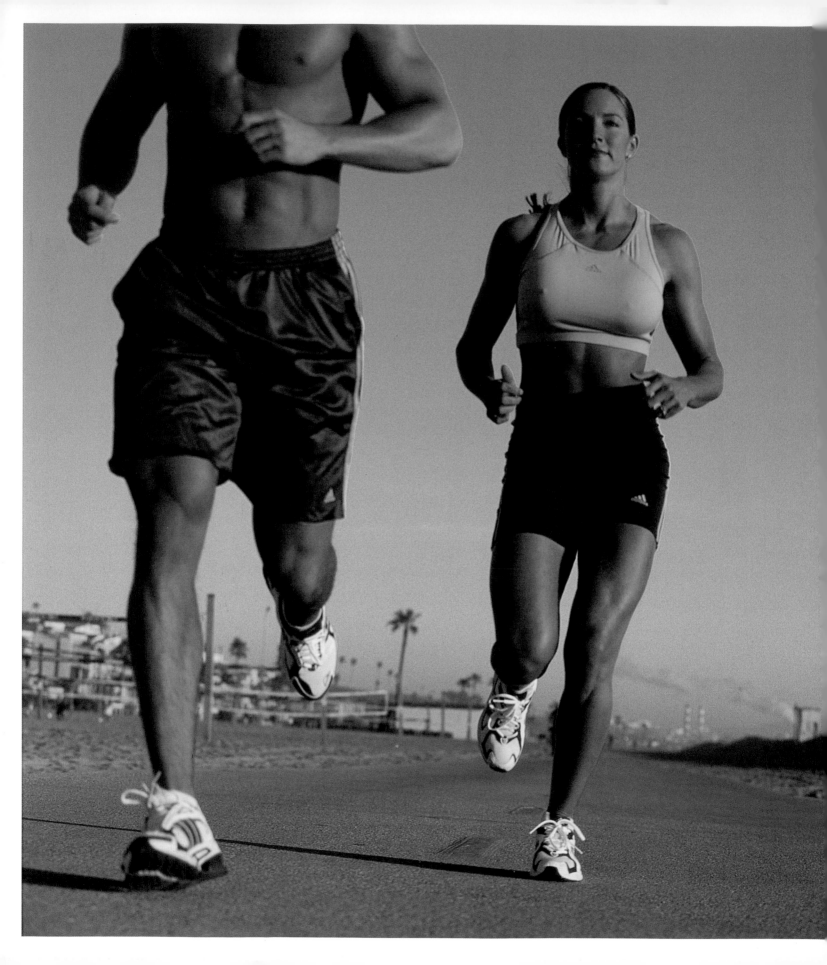

Go for the Burn

TRY THESE FOUR INTERVAL-TRAINING PROGRAMS TO SPEED UP YOUR FAT LOSS

Getting lean to show off your hard, muscular body means more than carefully watching your diet and dutifully training abs three times a week. If you seriously want to take your physique to the next level, you must do cardio regularly. While a leisurely ride on the recumbent bike is sure to burn a few calories, why not up the intensity and start melting away those love handles? That means work...and breaking out of your comfort zone. Sweat. Burning. Overloading your cardiovascular system, like how your weight workouts

overload your muscles. The same principles apply here, and turning up the intensity in your cardio training will provide the twin benefits of not only a leaner, more ripped physique but also improved aerobic fitness and heart health.

Unless you're a highly conditioned athlete, you won't be able to maintain a very intense pace for very long (as you approach your anaerobic threshold), so the best way to improve your aerobic fitness and burn fat is with intervals. That is, you alternate very intense periods of work with lower-intensity sessions in which you recover. (Your muscles eliminate lactic acid accumulation and use oxygen — hence the name aerobic — to carry out the lower-intensity metabolic processes.)

In a nutshell, you cycle periods of huffing and puffing with catching your breath, and then do it all over again. It won't be easy, but it sure breaks up the boredom of a long, constant-intensity workout, and you get all the benefits described above.

Exercise physiologists measure cardio training intensity with what's called age-related maximum heart rate (MHR). Though

MHR is an approximation, you can calculate it by subtracting your age from the number 220. An individual who's 30, then, has an MHR of 190. That's an estimate for the maximum number of times your heart can beat in a minute. Using either a heart-rate monitor or actually taking your pulse for 10 seconds and multiplying by 6 (for heart rate in beats per minute), you can manipulate your training to work in various training zones. Alternate zones, from high intensity to low intensity and back, and you're doing interval training.

Try these four interval-type programs, presented on the following pages, choosing which to do based on your aerobic fitness level. Feel free to shorten or lengthen them to suit your needs, but try to get at least 20 minutes of aerobic exercise in your target heart-rate zone at least three times a week. Bring the page with you to the gym or, if you work out at home, keep it handy while doing your cardio. Remember, the training-zone information works for any type of cardio (except the beginner's low-impact routine) and is a great tool to help you burn bodyfat and improve your level of aerobic fitness. So let's get ready to go for the burn!

Workout 1 — Beginner's Easy-Rider Low-Impact Workout (25 minutes)

This routine is designed to gradually elevate your heart rate without putting stress on your joints or connective tissue. This is ideal for those who aren't accustomed to regular aerobic exercise; the recumbent bike offers comfort and back support, and the elliptical trainer eliminates the repetitive jarring the joints are subjected to in a running program.

After you complete a five-minute warm-up, you'll work up to a slightly more intense pace, using that time to gradually bring your heart rate up to the target number. Maintain this pace, then switch pieces of equipment after five minutes. You'll slowly start to reduce the intensity to gradually reduce your heart rate and cool your body down on the elliptical trainer.

Note: *If you have only one piece of equipment, maintain the moderate heart-rate elevation for the full 16 minutes before beginning your cool-down.*

Workout 2 — Intermediate Fat-Zapper Workout (40 minutes)

During aerobic exercise, the body has two fuel options: carbohydrate, which is stored in the muscle as glycogen or in the blood as glucose; and/or fat, in the form of stored bodyfat or circulating fatty acids and triglycerides. While there has been some dispute as to what intensity of work is best for fat-burning, this interval routine allows you to reap the benefits of high- and moderate-intensity training simultaneously. While you do burn proportionately more fat than sugar (glycogen/glucose) at moderate intensities, you can burn a greater volume of fat at the higher intensities (total sugar usage will likely be higher as well).

As always, begin with a gradual warm-up. After you get your heart rate up, you simply alternate periods of high-intensity training with recovery intervals, each lasting two minutes. You'll need to determine which speed and/or resistance on your particular machine corresponds to the appropriate heart rate. Feel free to extend the recovery interval if necessary or push yourself a little longer when you can. As your endurance improves, you'll be able to sustain the higher-end elevations for longer periods. Strive to lengthen the high-intensity periods to up to five minutes, always alternating with two minutes of low-intensity recovery.

Workout 3 — Intermediate Graduated "Peak" Workout (30 minutes)

This intermediate workout pyramids up and down in intensity, rather than simply alternating high- and low-intensity intervals. Here, the middle of the session is the most intense, allowing for a continuous cool-down in stages.

After your warm-up, you'll go through three stages of intensity before working your way back down. In time, you can extend each of the intervals by a minute, bringing the entire exercise session to about 45 minutes.

Workout 4 — Advanced Fat-Burner Workout (35 minutes)

This program is for advanced exercisers who have already made challenging aerobic exercise a regular part of their fitness regimen. It can be incorporated with the other routines as a once-a-week all-out aerobic session to optimize fat-burning and endurance. Don't try this immediately before a weight-training session, as it may deplete your energy stores.

You're going to quickly work up to a high intensity and maintain it for as long as comfortably possible, cycling in short recovery periods that still keep your heart rate fairly elevated. Repeat these intervals several times before beginning your cool-down.

Intervals to Improve Aerobic Fitness & Fat-Burning

1) BEGINNER'S EASY-RIDER LOW-IMPACT WORKOUT (25 minutes)

Equipment: recumbent bike and elliptical trainer

DURATION (minutes)	DESCRIPTION	INTENSITY (THR)	INTENSITY (PE)
5	warm-up	50%	5
8	recumbent bike	65%	6-7
8	elliptical trainer	65%	6-7
4	cool-down	50%	5

2) INTERMEDIATE FAT-ZAPPER WORKOUT (40 minutes)

Equipment: your choice

DURATION (minutes)	DESCRIPTION	INTENSITY (THR)	INTENSITY (PE)
5	warm-up	50%	5
4	steady progress	60%	6
3	interval	70%	7
2	recovery	60%	6
2	interval	80%	8
2	recovery	60%	6
2	interval	80%	8
2	recovery	60%	6
2	interval	80%	8
2	recovery	60%	6
2	interval	80%	8
2	recovery	60%	6
2	interval	70%	7
3	recovery	60%	6
5	cool-down	50%	5

3) INTERMEDIATE GRADUATED "PEAK" WORKOUT (30 minutes)

Equipment: your choice

DURATION (minutes)	DESCRIPTION	INTENSITY (THR)	INTENSITY (PE)
5	warm-up	50%	5
3	steady progress	65%	6-7
1	higher intensity	75%	7-8
2	peak	85%	8-9
1	lower intensity	75%	7-8
2	recovery	65%	6-7
1	higher intensity	75%	7-8
2	peak	85%	8-9
1	lower intensity	75%	7-8
2	recovery	65%	6-7
1	higher intensity	75%	7-8
2	peak	85%	8-9
1	lower intensity	75%	7-8
2	recovery	65%	6-7
4	cool-down	50%	5

4) ADVANCED FAT-BURNER WORKOUT (35 minutes)

Equipment: your choice

DURATION (minutes)	DESCRIPTION	INTENSITY (THR)	INTENSITY (PE)
5	warm-up	50%	5
2	steady progress	70%	7
2	moderate-high intensity	80%	8
1	modest recovery	70%	7
1	high intensity	85%	8-9
2	modest recovery	70%	7
1	high intensity	85%	8-9
2	recovery	60%	6
1	high intensity	85%	8-9
2	modest recovery	70%	7
1	high intensity	85%	8-9
2	modest recovery	70%	7
1	high intensity	85%	8-9
2	modest recovery	70%	7
1	high intensity	85%	8-9
2	modest recovery	70%	7
2	low intensity	60%	6
5	cool-down	50%	5

Using Perceived Exertion to Gauge Intensity

Stopping your workout every couple of minutes to take your pulse is a ridiculous idea at best. If you don't have the benefit of using a heart-rate monitor, you can substitute perceived exertion (PE) for target heart rate (THR) to gauge the intensity of your cardio workouts. On a scale of 1–10, with 10 representing the highest level of intensity you can imagine, determine how hard you're working by how you feel. Conveniently, your THR and the PE numbers (1–10) correlate fairly closely, so if you feel you're working at about a 6 on the PE scale, you're most likely working at about 60% of your maximum heart rate.

Your Cardio Workout

The makeup of your aerobic training session should consist of three parts: warm-up (5–7 minutes), cardiovascular training session (20–40 minutes) and cool-down (4–7 minutes).

The warm-up serves to gradually prepare the working muscles, lungs and heart for the upcoming higher-intensity training. Warming up muscles, ligaments and tendons also reduces the chance of injury.

The actual training session ideally lasts for a minimum of 20 minutes, and to make improvements over time, you need to progressively overload your cardiovascular system to unaccustomed levels at least 2–3 times per week. Steady-state low-intensity workouts do little to increase aerobic fitness.

Cool down with another low-intensity stint to allow your working muscles and circulatory system to return to resting levels. Dropping the heart rate too quickly can cause dizziness and even fainting.

Good choices for aerobic activity are ones that include the body's largest muscle groups (most notably the legs and glutes) and can be maintained continuously.

Aerobic Training Guide

LEARN HOW TO UTILIZE YOUR HEART-RATE TRAINING ZONES

To work out at a safe and effective level, use target heart-rate training, which is essentially a measure of how hard you're working. By subtracting your age from 220, you get an approximation of your maximal heart rate. Based on your goals and experience level, work out in the appropriate zone during your training. Each zone is simply a percentage of your maximal heart rate. Immediately after slowing down, count your heart rate at your wrist or neck for 10 seconds and multiply that number by six (which provides your heart rate in beats per minute), or use a heart-rate monitor. Check to see which zone you fall into, and increase or decrease your intensity accordingly. Beginners should stick with the lower end of the range; check with your doctor before beginning any exercise program. Zones presented are predicted averages but may vary somewhat depending on your fitness level.

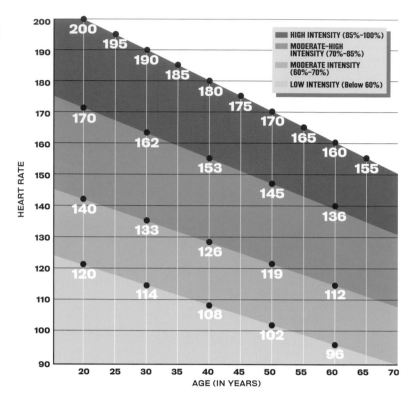

HIGH INTENSITY (85%–100%)
MODERATE–HIGH INTENSITY (70%–85%)
MODERATE INTENSITY (60%–70%)
LOW INTENSITY (Below 60%)

HEART RATE

AGE (IN YEARS)

Aerobic Training Zones Based on Target Heart Rate

LOW-INTENSITY ZONE

Training at or below 60% of your maximum heart rate (HR) may challenge novices but not those with high levels of cardiovascular fitness. It should feel fairly easy.
WHO SHOULD TRAIN IN THIS ZONE: This zone is ideal for warming up and cooling down, for advanced athletes recovering between high-intensity intervals and for beginners looking to get started on improving their aerobic fitness.
PREDOMINANT ENERGY SOURCES: Fat and blood glucose.
CALORIES BURNED: At this intensity level, you'll burn only a modest number of calories.

MODERATE/HIGH-INTENSITY ZONE

This is just below your anaerobic threshold, the level at which you cannot continue for long. Conditioned athletes train here to build above-average cardiovascular endurance and burn bodyfat. You know you're pushing yourself and have difficulty carrying on a conversation.
WHO SHOULD TRAIN IN THIS ZONE: Highly conditioned athletes and intermediates doing interval work.
PREDOMINANT ENERGY SOURCES: Muscle glycogen, and fat if you're a conditioned athlete.
CALORIES BURNED: You'll burn both more total calories and calories from fat than in lower-intensity levels.

MODERATE-INTENSITY ZONE

Elevating your HR to 60%–70% of your max delivers general health/cardio benefits, while burning more calories, including fat, than low-intensity training. You should be able to sustain this pace for extended periods, though you'll feel like you're working.
WHO SHOULD TRAIN IN THIS ZONE: Advanced beginners doing intervals, intermediates and athletes with superior fitness levels (as recovery stages during interval training).
PREDOMINANT ENERGY SOURCES: Fat, blood glucose and muscle glycogen.
CALORIES BURNED: Higher number than in the low-intensity zone.

HIGH-INTENSITY ZONE

You can't keep this pace up for more than several seconds. Well above anaerobic threshold (about 85% of your max HR or above), you fatigue quickly. You'll train here during some interval sessions but need to drop back down to recover. Builds speed and power.
WHO SHOULD TRAIN IN THIS ZONE: Very fit athletes and intermediates doing interval work for short periods.
PREDOMINANT ENERGY SOURCES: Muscle glycogen, muscle protein.
CALORIES BURNED: Because this type of training must be combined with lower-intensity levels during a particular workout, you maximize total calories burned while also burning bodyfat.

Adding Variety to Your Cardio Program

Choosing the same piece of cardio equipment each day not only leads to boredom but also increases the likelihood you'll hit a plateau. Change up your cardio activities instead, choosing a different exercise each day that you'll stick with through the entire workout. You can play with your intensity and duration variables, too, going longer and slightly easier on some days, shorter and more intense on others.

Here's a sample of how this routine might be applied by a more advanced athlete:

DAY	ACTIVITY	INTENSITY	DURATION
1	Stair-stepper	Low	40 minutes
2	Bicycle	High	20 minutes
3	Elliptical trainer	Intervals	30 minutes
4	Treadmill	Low	40 minutes
5	Rower	High	20 minutes
6	Your choice	Intervals	30 minutes
7	Rest		

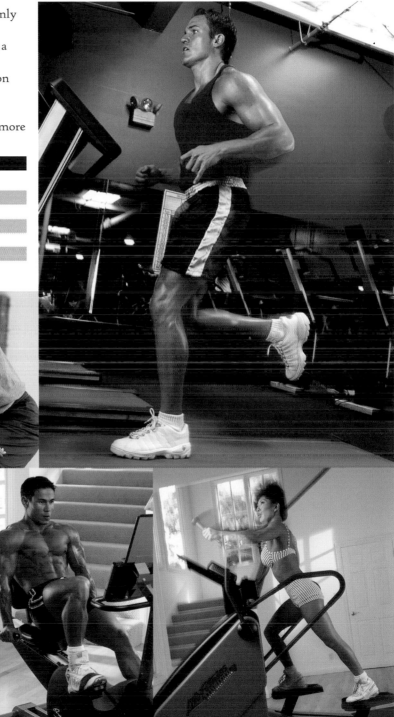

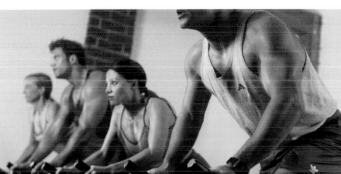

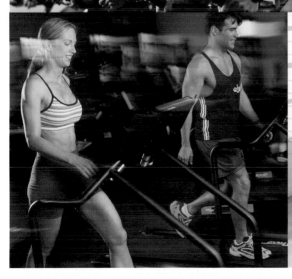

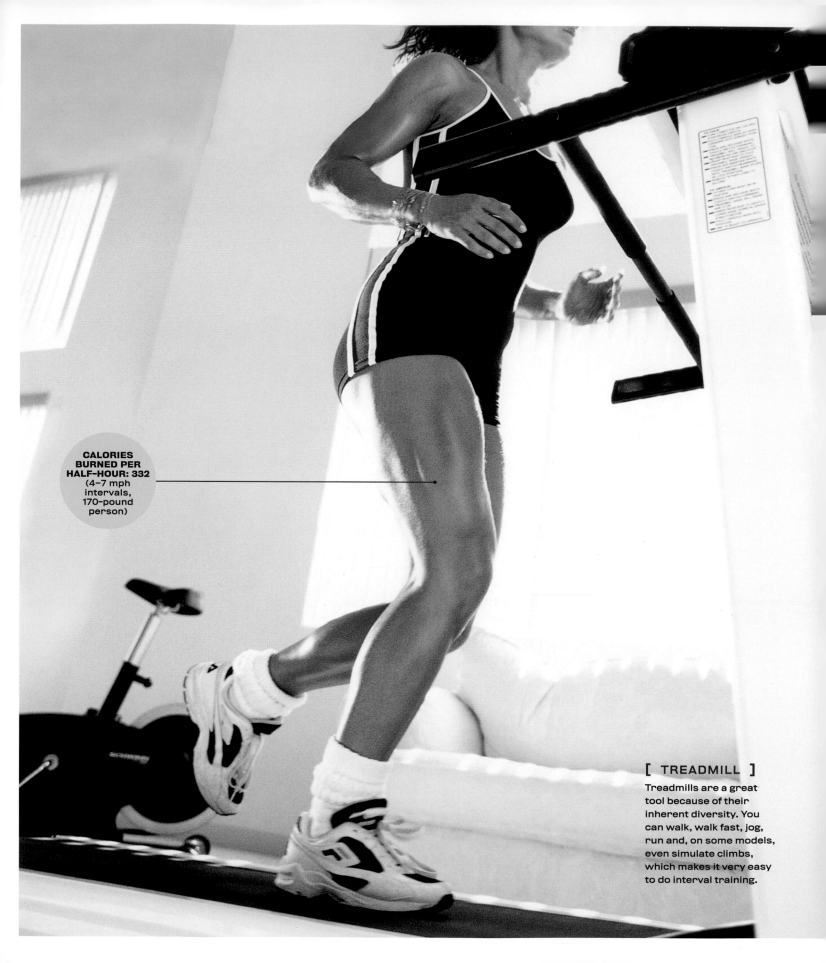

CALORIES BURNED PER HALF-HOUR: 332 (4–7 mph intervals, 170-pound person)

[TREADMILL]

Treadmills are a great tool because of their inherent diversity. You can walk, walk fast, jog, run and, on some models, even simulate climbs, which makes it very easy to do interval training.

Home Sweat Home

GET MORE FROM YOUR HOME CARDIO TRAINING WITH THESE **17 TIPS**

Working out at home can definitely be a challenge. Even if motivation isn't an issue, budgetary restraints on your home setup can make a heartpounding cardio session harder to achieve. But you really don't need a lot of high-tech gym equipment to meet your physique goals; instead, try our 17 economical options. And if you do have the budget for a piece of home cardio equipment, check out our reviews of the most popular pieces, from treadmills to indoor cycles, to help you make your purchasing decision.

1) Jump rope. About $5 can get you the simplest addition to your home gym. Think jumping rope is mere child's play? This metabolism-boosting workout can burn up to 742 calories per hour for a 160-pound person. A word of warning, however: This activity may be difficult to master, and you'll need to build up your endurance to be successful. Start slowly by jumping for 30 seconds, then running in place for 30 seconds. Add 15 seconds to your jump time until you can jump rope continuously for 10 minutes or longer.

2) Take the stairs. Whether you live in an apartment building, have a basement or work near a parking garage (stadium steps will also do, depending on the weather), stairs are a great way to incorporate interval training into your cardio regimen. Run up the stairs, then walk down, using that time for recovery. You could also use a step bench.

3) Use work-to-rest ratios to plan your interval training. For instance, use a ratio of 1:1 on your treadmill or elliptical trainer on Monday — one minute of sprinting to one minute of jogging. On Tuesday, up the recovery portion to two minutes so your work-to-rest ratio is 1:2 (one minute of sprinting to two minutes of jogging), which allows for a higher intensity work phase. The following day, return to the 1:1 ratio. Mixing things up taxes your energy systems differently in each workout and helps alleviate boredom.

4) Hit the video store. Home videos can be a welcome relief to hours spent on a stationary bike, mundane ab routines or flexibility training with no direction. Check out videos and DVDs from your local library, or purchase them from Wal-Mart, Target or online sources like www.bn.com, www.amazon.com or www.collagevideo.com. Some to try: *Aerobox* with Kathy Smith and 12-year boxing veteran Michael Olajide Jr. (1994, BodyVision); *Quick-Fix Tight Abs* with Minna

Lessig (2000, Peter Pan Studios); or *Embracing Power Yoga* with Mark Blanchard (1999, Spotlight Films). Check out www.videofitness.com for reviews on hundreds of videos, or log onto www.humankinetics.com for a huge selection of bodybuilding videos.

5) **Circuit train.** With your new jump rope, circuit training should be a breeze. You could do three supersets per bodypart, then jump rope for three minutes; jump rope or run in place for one minute between each superset; or do one set of a series of exercises, then perform 6–8 minutes of jumping rope or running in place between each series. All these options will get your heart rate up during your strength-training session.

6) **Use a heart-rate monitor.** For more efficient home cardio workouts, use a heart-rate monitor to make sure you're training in the appropriate target zones for your goals.

7) **Ride a bike.** Get on a stationary bike or turn your road bike into one. For $100–$300 you can purchase a cycling trainer that will elevate the back wheel of your bike or place both wheels on roller mechanisms so you can bike indoors. Unlike a stationary bike, using your own road bike will help you practice the balance associated with cycling and allow you to reach greater speeds. The only downfall? You can't create hilly terrain. Check out www.rei.com, www.aardvarkcycles.com or your local cycling store.

8) **Do sport drills** you used to hate from your high school football, basketball, soccer, baseball, wrestling or tennis days. By re-creating drills like line sprints, figure eights, agility drills and drop thrusts, you'll not only get a heart-pounding workout but alleviate boredom. Calisthenics like jumping jacks can also be worked into such a routine.

9) **Join a club.** If you're lacking the motivation to do some heavy breathing, a local training group may be the answer. Whether you choose to run, bike, swim, skate or almost anything else you can imagine, you'll have the opportunity to socialize with like-minded people. Internet sites like www.active.com and www.sportsmatchonline.com can help.

10) **Pump up the intensity** and make the time pass more quickly with music that gets you going. Jen Hendershott, 2004 Fitness Olympia runner-up, rotates her music and uses it to motivate her before a competition. Make tapes with your favorite tunes or use MP3 technology to create music mixes that match your workouts.

11) **Get everyone in on the act.** Sometimes our biggest deterrent to exercise is our family. Try making cardio activities a household affair — dancing to your favorite music, hiking or biking can involve all your loved ones.

12) **Make sure your garden grows.** "Planting a garden is a great way to burn calories and promote a healthy diet," remarks Cedric Bryant, PhD, senior vice president of sports medicine and research and development for StairMaster Health and Fitness Products, Inc. "All the standing, kneeling, walking, digging, weeding and watering can burn more than 400 calories an hour, and you'll reap a harvest of fresh vegetables for healthy eating."

13) **Design your own triathlon.** If you can't run, bike and swim, combine three other activities or cardio machines into one exercise session. With a rowing machine and stationary bike, for example, you can spend 10 minutes rowing, then run outside for 10 minutes, then jump on the stationary bike for 10 minutes. Break this up into mileage if you like.

14) **Play ball in the house.** Using a hacky-sack ball, bounce the ball off your knees, ankles and any other bodypart you can. Keep your knees high to elevate your heart rate. By trying to increase the number of uninterrupted repetitions you do, time will fly and your hand-eye coordination will soar.

15) **Get a hula hoop.** Man can't live by intense cardio alone. This inexpensive addition to your home gym will help promote flexibility and agility as well as back and abdominal strength. Or you can toss it on the ground and use it for agility drills.

16) **Jump into plyometrics.** When you incorporate bounding, jumping, throwing and other explosive movements into your routine, you'll stimulate increases in muscle growth and improve your athletic performance. For example, toss that hula-hoop on the ground, stand outside its circle and jump laterally into it. Immediately jump laterally out of it once you land, and repeat. You could also add a jump to your normal squat or play catch with a medicine ball.

17) **Park it.** Head to your local park or playground for a ton of fun cardio choices. Join a pickup basketball game. Ride the bike path or run the obstacle course. Hit the jungle gym for an upper-body workout. Do push-ups and crunches on the lawn. Run around the perimeter.

CALORIES BURNED PER HALF-HOUR: 323 (30–36 steps per 1-minute interval, 170-pound person)

CALORIES BURNED PER HALF-HOUR: 390 (moderate to high intensity, 170-pound person)

CALORIES BURNED PER HALF-HOUR: 334 (moderate- to high-intensity intervals, 170-pound person)

[HOME INDOOR CYCLE] (Spinning-type cycle)

(Above) The best way to power through an intense training session on your home indoor cycle is with music. Because this piece of machinery allows for many more positions and drills than a stationary bike, you can vary your workout and use music as the driving force behind what you do. Use fast songs for sprints and flats, medium-paced songs for jumps and walk/runs and slower songs for seated/standing climbs and jumps on hills.

[STAIR-STEPPER]

(Above left) If you have a stair-stepper at home, you can easily boost your workout to meet your high demands for intense training. But it won't be as intense if you lean into the handrails like you just finished a marathon. For added difficulty, you may want to use some lightweight dumbbells, since you can't increase resistance with the machine itself. Lay them on a table nearby so you can reach them easily. Hold one in each hand with elbows bent, in a kind of half hammer-curl position.

[ELLIPTICAL TRAINER]

(Left) The elliptical trainer is the newest kid on the cardio block and has been well-received. With great features like ramp and resistance control, preprogrammed courses and the ability to target certain muscle groups of the lower body, this cardio machine quickly crossed over from gym to home versions. Although quality and comfort differ from model to model, you can still get the most out of your trainer with interval training.

[CHAPTER SEVEN]

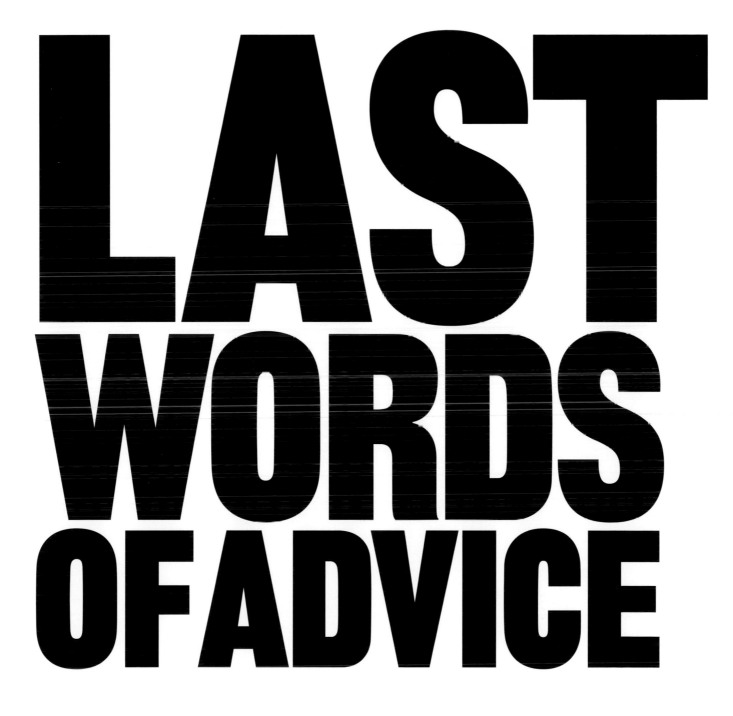

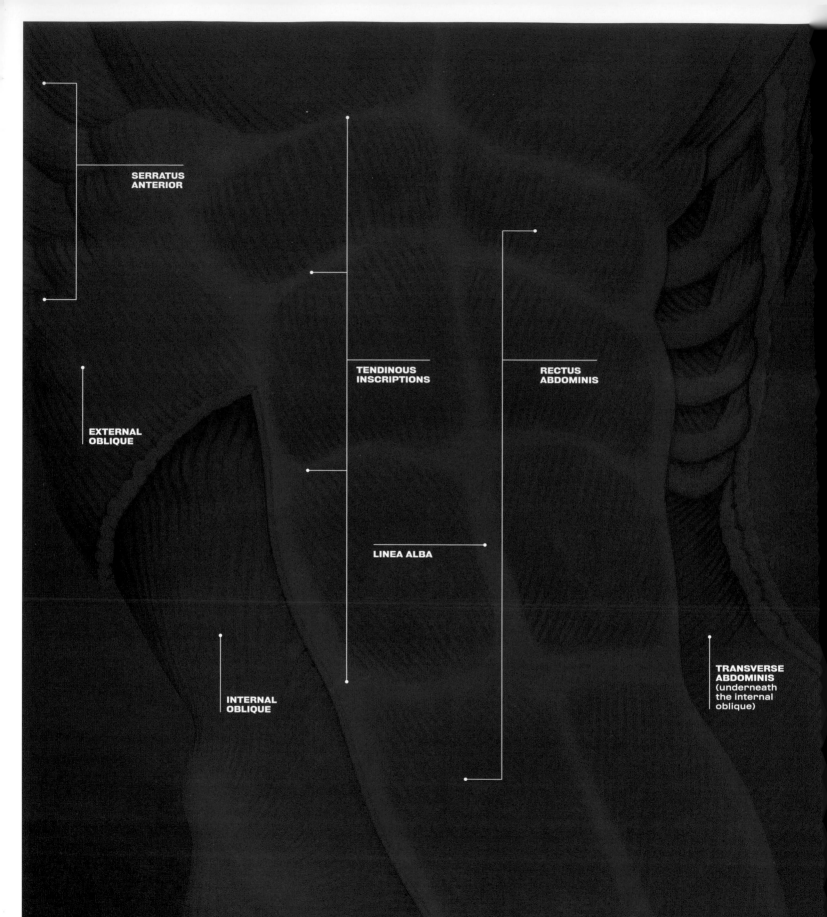

SERRATUS
ANTERIOR

EXTERNAL
OBLIQUE

INTERNAL
OBLIQUE

TENDINOUS
INSCRIPTIONS

LINEA ALBA

RECTUS
ABDOMINIS

TRANSVERSE
ABDOMINIS
(underneath
the internal
oblique)

Q&Abs

ANSWERS TO YOUR MOST COMMON QUESTIONS ABOUT YOUR MIDSECTION

During the first half of the '90s, a lot of sharp-if-otherwise-questionable "fitness gurus" made millions of dollars selling ab contraptions to American couch potatoes by promising that it took only minutes a day to lose years' worth of bodyfat. Though they gave us a good laugh, they underlined the value society seems to place on a washboard midsection and the amount of misinformation that's out there. If you're still striving for a six-pack, you should take heed of what you're about to read.

 Q: I train my abs religiously but can't seem to get the washboard look. What am I doing wrong?

A: There's more to ripped abs than blood, sweat and tears. You can have an extremely strong midsection, but it'll never show if it's buried beneath a layer of blubber. To get cut, you must eat right and increase your cardiovascular training, both of which will decrease bodyfat, making your abs more visible. Sure, genetics plays a role in body appearance and composition, but you can't reach your true potential without sound training and a low-fat diet.

Other factors to consider are training intensity, frequency and exercise selection. Just like any other muscle group, the abdominals require heavy resistance with a moderate number of repetitions to stimulate growth and size. Very high reps with light weights will give you a strong, supportive midsection, but won't lead to thicker abs.

Overtraining of the abdominal muscles is common, so if you're doing ab work daily, you need to cut back. Limit your ab training to three sessions per week, max. Additionally, you must find the exercises that work best for you and that target the main areas of the torso: upper- and lower-ab regions and obliques. Movements such as the crunch and reverse crunch are simple yet effective at shifting emphasis in your upper- and lower-ab regions, while adding a slight twisting motion to these exercises will effectively target your obliques.

Q: I've been thinking about buying one of those ab machines advertised on TV, but my training partner says they're worthless. What's the bottom line?

A: Actually, nothing is wrong with the majority of ab machines on the market. Generally speaking, they put your body in a good mechanical position and often provide lower-back support. Yet you can achieve the same results and train your abs just as well without machines or gimmicks. Learn how to properly execute each exercise, then determine which ones work best for you.

Q: The people I lift with at the gym train their abs daily, but I've read that you shouldn't train abs more than three times a week. Is this muscle group different from others?

A: In most respects, the abdominal muscles are the same as any other muscle group in the body and should be trained accordingly. Unlike most major muscles, however, the abs are almost always in a state of contraction as they work to maintain good posture (both in daily activities and in the gym). For this reason, the abdominals have a greater endurance component than most muscle groups, which may explain why they're often trained more frequently with higher repetitions.

If your goal is to have a strong midsection with good muscle tone, then use moderate resistance to perform about 20 reps per set. If you want thicker abs with noticeable peaks and valleys, you must stick to a traditional regimen of heavy resistance with a lower number of repetitions. Choose a resistance or an exercise that allows you to do 10–12 repetitions (which is slightly higher than for other bodyparts). The last couple of reps should be difficult and cause a burning sensation in the abdominal region.

If you're a beginner, start with one exercise each for the lower- and upper-ab regions and obliques. Perform 2–3 sets of each exercise with about a minute's rest between sets. As your training and strength progress, add another exercise per region and decrease the amount of rest between sets to 20–30 seconds. Regardless of whether you're training for size or tone, limit your ab training to three sessions or fewer per week. It may feel as though your abdominal muscles recuperate faster than other muscle groups, but they still need that much rest to grow bigger and stronger.

Q: I know that choosing the right exercises is important to build a strong midsection, but how critical is the order in which you perform them?

A: Though the answer to this question is subject to debate, many experts recommend that the lower-abdominal area should be trained before the upper region and obliques. The lower abs are generally the weakest region, due in part to less-frequent training but largely because of the involvement of the hip flexors that assist with many lower-abdominal movements. Additionally, the obliques and upper abs are needed to stabilize and immobilize the upper body during lower-ab training, so they need to be fresh and strong to ensure that you can maintain proper form (which wouldn't happen if you do upper abs first). Good form for lower-ab movements means minimal hip-flexor movement and maximal contraction of the lower abdominal region.

Once your lower-ab strength is on par with the rest of your midsection muscles, you can experiment with the order in which you train your various ab muscles. Work the upper region first one day, obliques first the next and the lower region first in your last ab session of the week. Another strategy that works especially well for your abs is supersets. Perform one set of lower-ab movements, followed immediately by a set for upper abs and a set for obliques. Remember, variety is not only the spice of life but it's also the golden rule of growth for bodybuilding.

Q: Is the abdominal muscle a single muscle or a group of related muscles?

A: The abdominals are a collective group of muscles that includes the rectus abdominis, external obliques, internal obliques and transverse abdominis. They all work together to stabilize your torso, provide support for your spinal column and facilitate movement at your waist.

Even though it appears to be a six-pack of muscles on someone who's massive and ripped, the rectus abdominis is a single muscle that runs vertically from the pelvis up to the ribs. Because of its great length, a distinction is usually made between the upper and lower regions. The regions cannot be isolated, but emphasis can be shifted from one end to the other by choosing the appropriate exercise. In general, the upper-ab region is best stimulated by securing your lower body and flexing your torso (as you do in the crunch). The opposite is true for lower-abdominal training: Secure your upper body and bring your legs and pelvis up (as you do in the reverse crunch).

You should note that the transverse abdominis isn't visible and causes little movement, so it's rarely the focus of any training program.

Q: Everyone talks about eliminating the hip flexors when training abs. Why is this important, and how would I do it?

A: Eliminating the hip flexors when performing abdominal exercises is important for one simple reason: to emphasize and provide maximal stimulation to the ab muscles, not the hip flexors. Doing so, however, isn't always such a simple task.

Both the hip flexors and rectus abdominis cross the hip joint and are the prime movers in hip flexion. The hip flexors are most involved when your feet are secured — even if your knees are bent — and when you fully extend your legs and hips (such as when you lie flat on your back). If you bring your knees to your chest from an extended lying position, the hip flexors initially do most of the work. But as your knees come closer to your chest, the hip flexors begin to give way to the lower abdominal muscles as you rotate your pelvis. The lower abs reach maximal contraction and the hip flexors call it quits by the time your knees reach your chest.

IN MOST RESPECTS, YOUR AB MUSCLES ARE THE SAME AS ANY OTHER MUSCLE GROUP IN YOUR BODY, AND THEY SHOULD BE TRAINED ACCORDINGLY

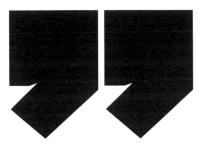

Keep your knees bent and unsecured to minimize hip-flexor involvement when performing abdominal exercises. Also keep in mind that you can never totally isolate your abdominals; some hip-flexor activation will always be present.

Q: I've heard that abdominal strength is important for a healthy back, but what's the connection?

A: The midsection, or torso, of the human body is the center of support and stability for the entire upper body, especially the spinal column. The abdominal muscles, coupled with the muscles of the lower back, provide a natural brace for the spine and hold it securely in place. Contraction of the abdominal muscles causes increased intra-abdominal pressure, which in turn provides the support necessary to keep the spine in proper alignment. Without adequate support, heavy weight-bearing exercises become potentially more dangerous. The possibility of disc misalignment or slippage rises as the forces placed upon them increase. Even if no acute pain is evident, repetitive trauma to the spinal column can eventually lead to injury.

Q: I've noticed that many of the pros and advanced bodybuilders say they train their abs infrequently. How can they get by with such minimal ab training?

A: These athletes have paid their dues by spending countless hours pumping iron and developing their physiques. Although room for improvement always exists, the abdominal area often develops quickly and subsequently needs less training. Too much ab work, in fact, can excessively build the midsection, especially the obliques, which can detract from overall body symmetry and make the waist wider, ruining the pleasing V-shaped physique. Bottom line, most pros no longer want to build up this bodypart.

Q: I've just returned to training after a low-back injury. Do you have any advice regarding ab training to prevent aggravation or re-injury? Should I avoid certain exercises?

A: Proper form is always important when exercising, but it's especially critical when you're coming off an injury. The key to avoiding or preventing back pain is maintaining a neutral alignment of the spinal column at all times, particularly when exercising but also during normal, daily activities. Neutral alignment is achieved by keeping the natural "S" contour of the spine, without excessive arching or flattening of the back. With a properly aligned spine, the ears, shoulders, hips, knees and ankles will form a perfectly straight line when viewed from the side. This neutral position provides optimal load distribution and minimal stress to the vertebrae and discs of the spine.

To prevent re-injury, stick with basic abdominal movements — crunches and reverse crunches — remembering to maintain the spine's neutral alignment. Lynette Dèry, PT, a physical therapist at Progressive Step Rehabilitation Services in Jacksonville, Florida, says: "Imagine that your midsection is in a cast, preventing your back from arching or bending. This will help maintain proper spinal alignment and reduce the forces applied to the discs." Although this rigid body position may appear to limit your ability to achieve maximal contraction, your ab training won't suffer and neither will your back. If you've been injured, forget about any twisting or side-bending movements, as they'll only place excessive forces on your discs.

Contraindicated exercises for low-back injuries include any sit-up (feet anchored or free), the cross-knee crunch and variations of the hanging leg raise. In fact, avoid any abdominal exercises that prevent you from bending your knees. In the full-range sit-up, the chest travels all the way up to the knees. Abdominal contraction nears its peak as the shoulder blades come off the ground during the ab crunch, so you don't need to continue the movement. After 30–45 degrees, keeping your back in neutral alignment becomes impossible. The farther you come up, the more your back bends and the more stress is placed on the lumbar and thoracic discs.

Dèry recommends not using a crunch machine that forces you into a 90-degree upright sitting position. She explains: "Studies have shown that the sitting position alone loads the discs. Forward bending while sitting (especially with weight attached) puts a tremendous amount of pressure on the discs of your lower back." Good choices for ab work would include crunches and bent-leg raises without anchored feet.   *(See references on page 164)*

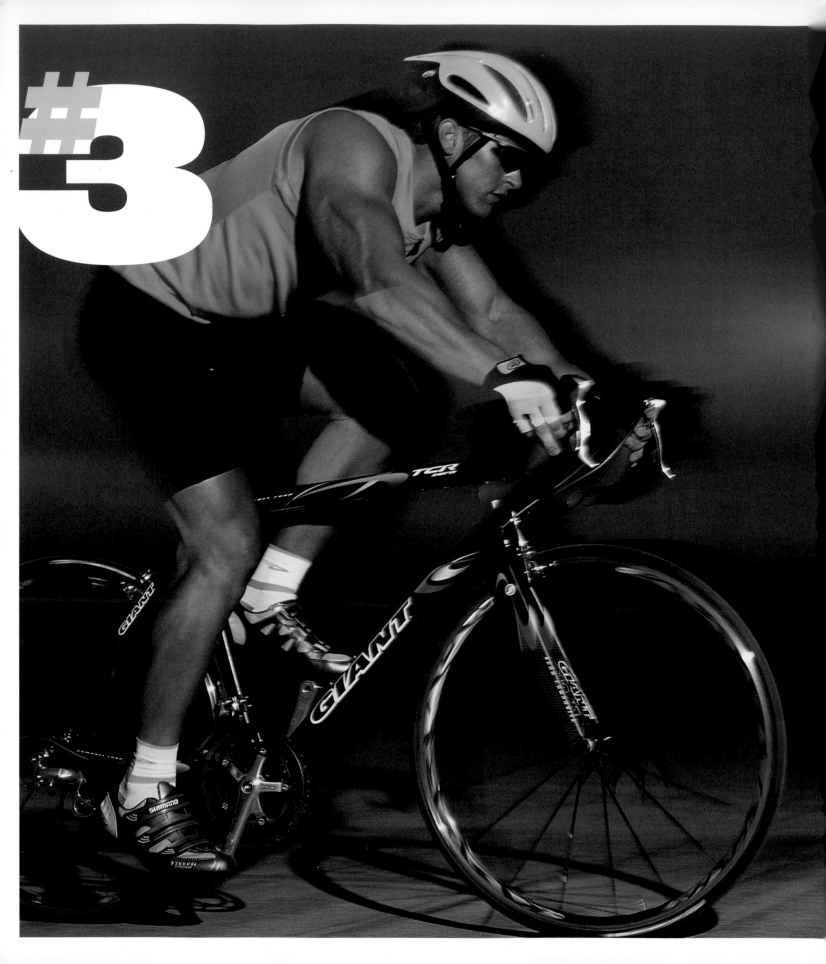

Middle Management

USE THESE **31 TIPS** TO BRING OUT YOUR ABS AND SHED BODYFAT FOR GOOD

Losing fat is a tricky thing. Sadly, we can't give you just one answer to reverse years of late-night beer runs, fast-food binges and liberal use of salad dressings. We did, however, come up with 31 ways to give bodyfat a proper send-off. A significant part of it has to do with your lifting and cardio regimens, which we address here. Another big part takes place in the kitchen and during the rest of your day, so we also present a practical list for cleaning up your eating habits and, as a result, your physique.

[LIFESTYLE]

1) Change your lifestyle

When you go on a "program" to lose bodyfat, you may set yourself up for failure. A program implies an endpoint, which is when most people return to their previous habits. *If you want to lose fat and keep it off, make changes that you can live with indefinitely.* Don't over-restrict calories, and find an exercise program that adequately challenges you, provides progression and offers sufficient variety so you can maintain it for years to come.

2) Know how to weigh yourself

The bathroom scale is a valuable tool for monitoring fat loss — if you really know how to use it. Since bodyweight can radically change throughout the day and from day to day, weigh yourself each morning upon rising and keep an eye out for "lower lows." *Look for the scale to nudge* lower two days out of every 10. If this is the case, you're reducing your bodyweight. If you fail to hit a new lower bodyweight twice every 10 days, adjust your caloric intake or increase your caloric expenditure by exploring more of the diet tips listed here.

3) Don't be lazy

You've heard it a million times, but it's worth repeating: Don't be lazy! *When looking for a parking space at the mall, park far away from the door so you have to walk farther.* Use the stairs instead of the elevator or escalator. Don't use the self-propel mode of your lawnmower when mowing your yard. Ride your bike or walk when possible, instead of driving your car.

4) Suck in that gut

An athlete tip that has some theoretical base but is without research is to suck in your gut. Several intra-abdominal muscles are responsible for pulling your abdominal wall inward, and *by continuously contracting these muscles (holding the fully contracted position and repeating), you may be able to condition them to remain shortened.* Many athletes swear by this as a way to decrease the appearance of an outward-protruding gut. Feel free to give it a try.

[NUTRITION]

5) Drink more water

Water is the medium in which most cellular activities take place, including the transport and burning of fat. In addition, drinking plenty of calorie-free water makes you feel full and eat less. *Drink at least 1 ounce of water per 2 pounds of bodyweight a day* (that's 100 ounces for a 200-pound person). Keep a 20-ounce water bottle at your desk, fill it five times a day and you're set.

6) Reduce starchy carbs

Consuming too many starchy foods, such as potatoes, rice, pasta and breads (especially in one sitting) provides your body with more than it needs for energy and glycogen stores; anything left over will be stored as fat. "You don't have to eliminate starchy carbs completely," says IFBB pro bodybuilder Mike Matarazzo. "But you should really cut back on them when trying to shed bodyfat." *Limit total starch servings per day to 3–5, with a serving size being 1 cup of pasta, rice or sliced potatoes.*

7) Limit sugar consumption

Taking in simple carbs (sugars) right after weight training replenishes muscle and liver glycogen stores, but excess sugar consumed at other times will be stored as fat. Satisfy your sweet tooth occasionally, but try limiting your intake of sugar to fresh fruit. *Replace sugary beverages like soft drinks and juice with water, coffee, teas or diet soda.*

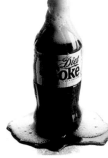

8) Eat the proper amount of protein

Many bodybuilders jack their protein consumption through the roof when they diet. But protein has calories, too, which can be stored as fat if overconsumed. *Take in 1–1.5 grams of protein per pound of bodyweight each day* (200–300 grams for a 200-pound person). This provides a sufficient amount of amino acids to maintain muscle mass, while keeping your total calorie count under control.

9) Eat a full, balanced breakfast

"Your body has been starving all night long, and it needs nutrients to rebuild itself," advises Mike. "If you just catch something quick on the run instead of eating a full meal, it negatively impacts your workout and everything else you do during the day." *Eat sufficient protein (30–40 grams), a complex carbohydrate like oatmeal and a piece of fruit to start your day off right.*

10) Cut calories by 10%–15%

The energy equation in weight loss is generally a pretty simple concept: Eat less and you'll lose weight. Yet some people go overboard and severely cut back on their caloric intake, which can cause a drop in energy levels and hinder efforts in the gym. Worse, big calorie cuts can slow metabolism as the body adapts to a lower energy intake. *More moderate cuts will cause the burning of stored bodyfat while allowing you to train with maximal effort.* If you eat 3,000 calories a day, drop to between 2,700 and 2,550 calories a day.

11) Avoid drastic calorie reductions

"Any competitor who drastically cuts calories to try to get leaner for a show learns that's not the best way to do it," notes IFBB fitness competitor Laurie Vaniman. "You end up looking flat and depleted." The same holds true for noncompetitors; aim for a modest decrease in calories instead. *Smaller bodybuilders shouldn't cut more than 200–300 calories per day, and larger bodybuilders shouldn't cut more than 500,* says nutrition expert and former bodybuilder Chris Aceto.

12) Increase vegetable consumption

Vegetables are nutrient-dense, meaning they pack maximum nutrition value with minimal calories, leaving you fuller on fewer calories. *Consume five servings of veggies a day* — as a snack, on a sandwich or on the side of a chicken breast. Order your next burger with fresh vegetables instead of french fries.

13) Consume 25–35 grams of fiber a day

"Fiber lowers insulin levels — along with total calories — affecting how lean you'll get," says Aceto. Fiber absorbs water and takes up more space in your stomach, which helps fight off hunger pangs. *Some great sources of fiber include bran cereal, oatmeal and beans.* Check nutrition labels for fiber content.

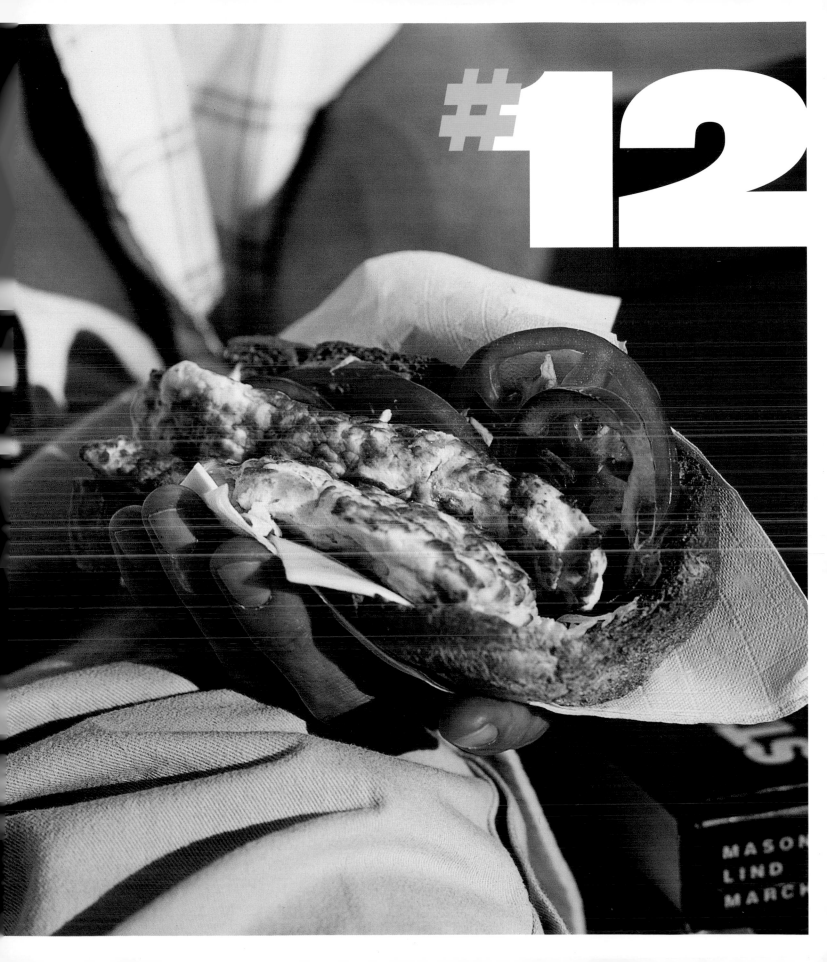

#12

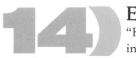

Eat more healthy fats

"Healthy fats are totally underutilized by individuals trying to shed bodyfat," remarks Mike. "You have to reduce calories to get rid of bodyfat, but you don't want to cut out healthy fats completely." Fats take longer to break down in your stomach and help control blood-sugar levels, leaving you more satisfied and reducing your cravings. *Include avocados, fatty fish, olives, nuts and seeds and oils such as olive, flaxseed and canola in your diet.*

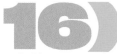

Spice things up

Red peppers, the spicy ingredient in many ethnic dishes, contain capsaicin, which can increase your metabolic rate when taken with meals. Don't expect any major miracles, but *spiking your chicken dishes with red peppers might provide a slight increase in whole-body thermogenesis.* Alternatively, you can gulp 5–10 encapsulated grams of capsaicin from your local health-food store.

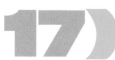

Take your multivitamin/ mineral and antioxidants

Even though a healthy meal plan probably contains the RDA for most of your recommended vitamins and minerals each day, you'd be smart to *consume at least one multi in the morning with breakfast.* As an added measure of protection against oxidative stress related to a negative calorie balance and high training intensities, consume supplemental vitamins E and C in the morning and evening (approximately 500 IUs and 2 grams, respectively, per day.)

[EXERCISE]

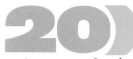

If you're training other bodyparts, do most of your ab work afterward

If you're performing a routine for another part of your body and you plan to do abs as well, you might want to begin your workout with a few minutes of ab moves to stimulate your body's core and prepare it for the training ahead. However, *you should save most of your abdominal exercises for the end of your workout.* You don't want to overly fatigue your midsection before you ask it to support a dynamic movement like squats, rows or lunges. If you choose to train your abs first (which is a good idea if you tend to get tired at the end of your workouts and blow them off), consider exercising them on days when you have less need for stabilization (such as when working chest, shoulders or arms).

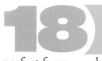

Don't overtrain

Doing more is not necessarily better. In reality, 30 crunches done slowly and with perfect form — where you contract your abs strongly on every rep — are better than 100 crunches done poorly. *In training, there comes a point of diminishing returns: When you push your body too hard and for too long, you actually lose muscle tissue while the fat stays put.* If you work hard for 20–30 minutes in an ab workout, don't think another 30 minutes will get you that much closer to your goal. In this game, quality and consistency are more valuable than quantity.

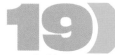

Don't train your abs every day

Abs have the same fast- and slow-twitch muscle fibers as the other muscles of your body. So, like other muscles, you can't train them every day and expect them to recover adequately. However, unlike other muscles, they do tend to recover pretty quickly, so *training them every other day to every third day is smart.*

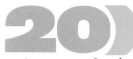

Push yourself a little further each time

When you train, your body adapts by getting stronger. *In order to keep making gains in your muscle strength and fitness levels, you have to keep challenging yourself.* For example, if you can do 15 reps of crunches, try for 16–17 per set next time. Or you can try other things to increase the difficulty level, like doing your reps more slowly or choosing a slightly harder exercise. Over the course of weeks and months, you'll find that you're able to do things you never would've imagined on your first day of training.

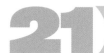

Train your abs for endurance, not growth

If your goal is to have a slimmer waistline, don't train your abs with heavy loads. Use a weight that allows you to get at least 15 reps per set, allowing minimal rest between sets (less than 60 seconds). Or use only your own bodyweight as resistance while maximally contracting your abs on each and every repetition.

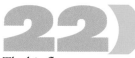

Be careful to keep your hip flexors from taking over in your ab workouts

The hip flexors are powerful muscles that run alongside your hips, and they can sometimes dominate an exercise in which you're trying to work your abs. Although completely preventing

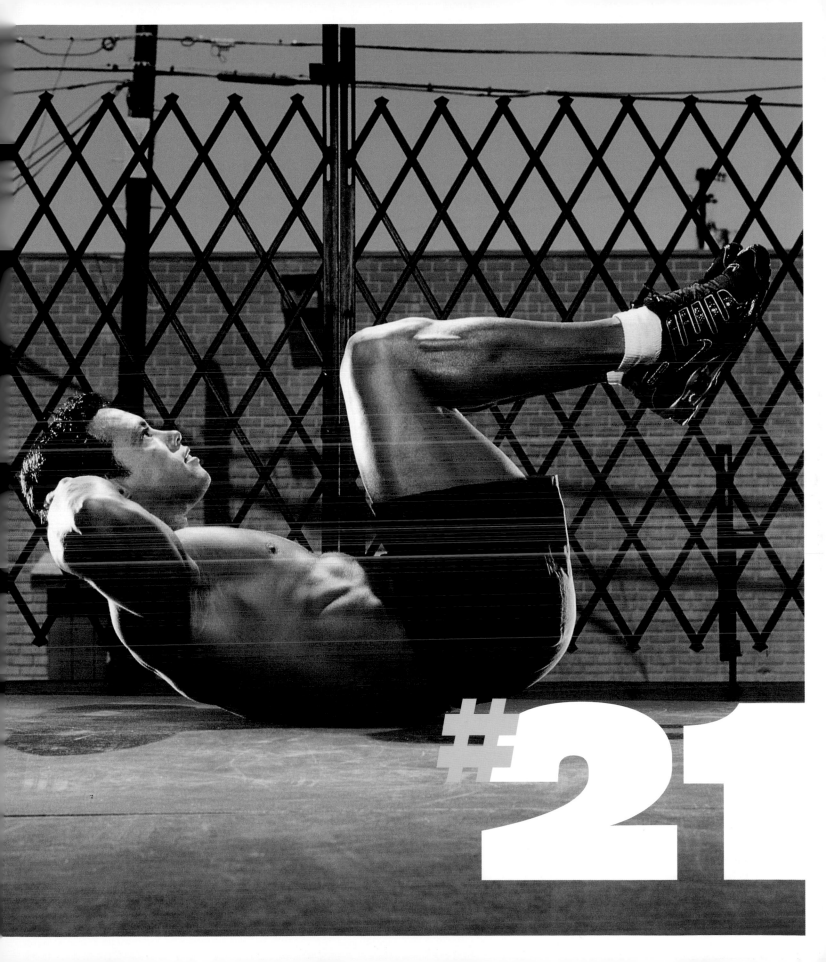

#21

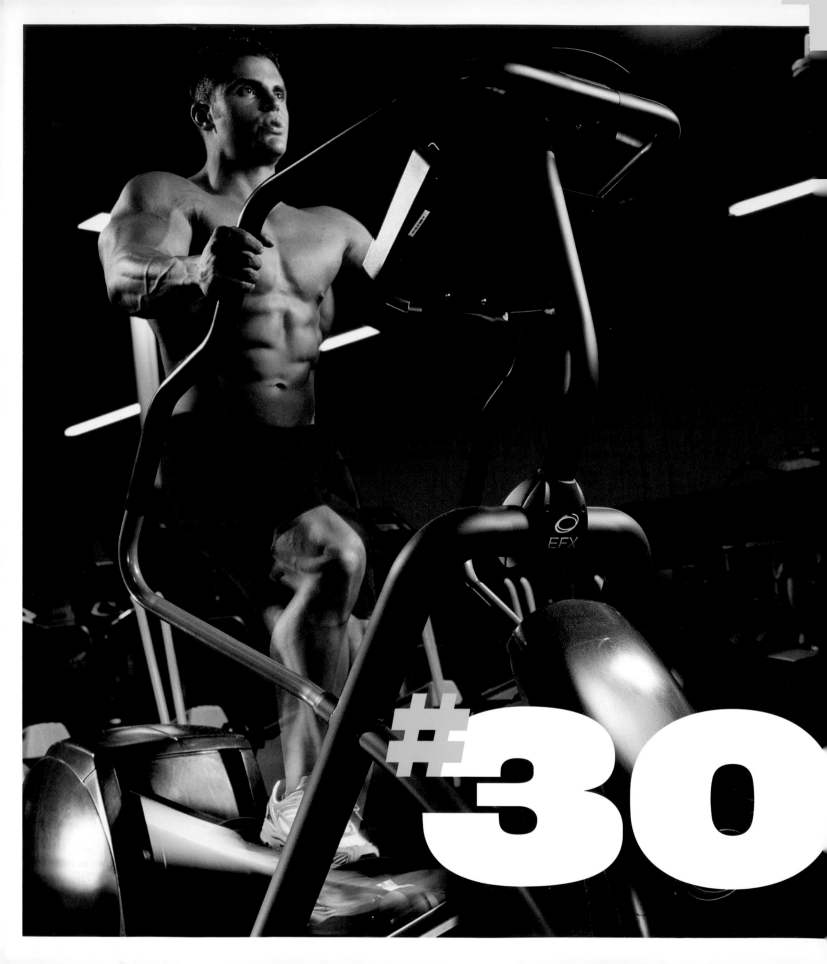

#30

the hip flexors from working is probably impossible, good technique can diminish their involvement. *Make sure your ab moves take place at the spine (it should curl on a crunch, for example), and not at your hips.* Also, many beginners often put their feet under a bar or have a friend hold their feet to the ground while they do sit-ups or crunches, but that enables the body to curl up without any big effort from the abs if your form is sloppy. If you choose anchored ab exercises (like decline-bench crunches, for example), perform them after doing nonanchored moves.

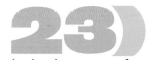

Variety is good

Once you've mastered the basic exercises and built a solid foundation (such as by using our five-week plan in Chapter 2 of this book), add different exercises to your program. *Choosing a variety of moves serves two purposes: It "shocks" the muscles, preventing them from becoming accustomed to the same exercise, and it helps you stress the muscles from different angles, maximizing your returns by ensuring that you stimulate more of your middle area.*

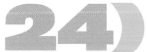

Keep your low back strong

Virtually every muscle group in your body has an opposing muscle group that needs to be trained for balance (for example, your biceps and triceps in your arms or your quadriceps and hamstrings in your thighs). The antagonist to your abs is your lower back. *To prevent an imbalance of strength that could lead to pain or injury, work the lower back muscles regularly* with back extensions or even deadlifts (if you train regularly with weights).

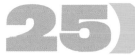

Train like a bodybuilder to help improve your hormonal milieu

Doing 3–5 sets of 8–12 reps with relatively short rest periods (1–2 minutes) has been shown to increase testosterone and growth hormone release, improving your anabolic environment and metabolism.

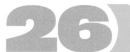

Choose compound movements

Burn more calories by selecting the highly demanding exercises that require the most muscle mass to complete. Examples include squats, bent-over rows, presses for chest or shoulders, deadlifts, etc. Exercises that involve only one muscle group (such as biceps curls, leg extensions, triceps pressdowns) don't require as much energy. *Make compound movements the backbone of your weight-training workout.*

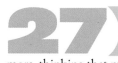

Go heavy

A lot of people make the mistake of using very light weights for 15 reps or more, thinking that more reps will help burn more calories and bodyfat. In reality, that's a very inefficient way to train. Muscle tissue burns fat, and *the best way to build muscle is with sets of 8–12 reps, using a weight heavy enough that it challenges you to finish each set.*

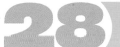

Evaluate your progress regularly

Who does the same thing over and over again, hoping for a different result? An idiot! Don't be one. *If, after a month or two on this or any other training program, positive changes to your body aren't taking shape, stop and rethink your strategy.* Your body will adapt and change, and you can add muscle while losing fat — but you need a dedicated, precise strategy to make it happen. Don't settle for zero progress; putting yourself through a strict diet and tough workouts week after week isn't worth the effort and sacrifice if you're not reaching your goals.

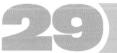

Don't daydream when you train

Concentrate on each contraction of your muscles during every single repetition you perform. No magic number of reps exists that equals a great midsection, so don't just go blindly for a set goal in your head; *do each rep as if it was the most important, because at that moment, it is.*

[CARDIO]

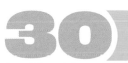

Push harder or longer to continually boost your metabolism

As with weight training, your muscles also learn to adapt to your cardio training. Therefore, to continuously see improvement in your level of cardiovascular health and ability to oxidize fats and carbs, *you need to progressively push your training above its current limitations.* This can be accomplished by simply adding a minute to your workout, increasing the incline on a treadmill or working at a higher maximum rate.

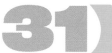

Maximize your metabolism

According to scientific evidence, *men may benefit from doing cardio for longer durations and lower relative intensities* (approximately 65% of max heart rate). *Women may see better overall benefits by exercising at higher levels of intensity,* such as interval training, to burn significantly more overall calories and fat.

[REFERENCES]

The Zigzag Diet

(Continued from page 125)

>> Di Pasquale, M. Amino acids and proteins for the athlete: the anabolic edge. New York, NY: CRC Press, 1997.

>> Dulloo, A.G., Calokatisa, R. Adaptation to low calorie intake in obese mice: contribution of a metabolic component to diminished energy expenditure during and after weight loss. International Journal of Obesity 15:7–16, 1991.

>> Forbes, G.B., et al. Hormonal response to overfeeding. American Journal of Clinical Nutrition 49(4):608–611, 1989.

>> Maughan, R.J., et al. Diet composition and the performance of high-intensity exercise. Journal of Sport Science 15(3):265–275, 1997.

>> Nair, K.S., et al. Leucine, glucose and energy metabolism after 3 days of fasting in healthy human subjects. American Journal of Clinical Nutrition 46(4):57–562, 1987.

>> Rothwell, J., et al. Hormonal and metabolic responses to fasting and refeeding. International Journal of Obesity 9(Suppl 2):49–54, 1985.

>> Roy, H.J., et al. Substrate oxidation and energy expenditure in athletes and nonathletes consuming isoenergetic high- and low-fat diets. American Journal of Clinical Nutrition 67(3):405–411, 1998.

>> Saris, W.H. Effects of energy restriction and exercise on the sympathetic nervous system. International Journal of Obesity and Related Metabolic Disorders 19(Suppl 7):S17–S23, 1995.

One Week to Peak

(Continued from page 132)

>> Bowtell, J.L., et al. Effects of oral glutamine on whole body carbohydrate storage during recovery from exhaustive exercise. Journal of Applied Physiology 86(6):1,770–1,777, 1999.

Q & Abs

(Continued from page 155)

>> Axler, C., McGill, S. Low back loads over a variety of abdominal region exercises: searching for the safest abdominal challenge. Medicine & Science in Sports & Exercise 29(6):804–811, 1997.

>> Halpern, A.A., Bleck, E.E. Sit-up exercises: an electromyographic study. Clinical Orthopaedics Nov–Dec (145):172–178, 1979.

>> Nachemson, A.L. Disc pressure measurements. Spine Jan-Feb 6(1):93–97, 1981.